RYAN BLUMENTHAL

AUTOPSY

*Life in the trenches with a
forensic pathologist in Africa*

Jonathan Ball Publishers

Johannesburg ● Cape Town ● London

© Text: Ryan Blumenthal 2020
© Cover image: iStock / Image Source
© Photo on the back cover: Elmi de Pauw / Walla Films
© Published edition: Jonathan Ball Publishers 2020

Originally published in South Africa in 2020 by
JONATHAN BALL PUBLISHERS
A division of Media24 (Pty) Ltd
PO Box 33977, Jeppestown, 2043

This edition published in 2021 by Jonathan Ball Publishers
An imprint of Icon Books Ltd, Omnibus Business Centre,
39-41 North Road, London N7 9DP
Email: info@iconbooks.com
For details of all international distributors, visit iconbooks.com/trade

ISBN 978-1-77619-110-9
e-ISBN 978-1-77619-019-5

Printed and bound in Great Britain
by Clays Ltd, Elcograf S.p.A.

Dedicated to all the heroes
who practise forensics in Africa.
You know who you are.

Contents

Introduction

Even though they cannot speak, the dead have a lot to say. The moment you realise this, you have understood one of the first cornerstones of forensic pathology.

A second cornerstone is the instruction to question everything. Why does the gunshot victim have a specific kind of tattoo? What is under the female rape victim's fingernails? Why are the businessman's teeth in such bad condition?

A forensic pathologist is a qualified medical doctor – that is, someone who is technically, physically, emotionally and psychologically equipped to examine the dead. Forensic pathologists, also known as medical examiners in countries like the USA, look for clues on a dead body. To them, a dead body is a crime scene of sorts.

Forensic pathologists investigate medicolegally significant – in other words, questionable – deaths, and try to bring closure to the deceased's next of kin by establishing, among other things, the cause of death. We serve justice and not the police or prosecution, both of whom have a responsibility to prove beyond reasonable doubt that a crime has been committed. Forensic pathologists help bring perpetrators to justice or exonerate the innocent. Without good legal medicine, there cannot be justice. Although there are differences in forensic medicine between countries, its philosophy has always remained the same: it was born from the need for justice. So, while there are valuable lessons to be learnt from the dead, this book is written for the living.

As a forensic pathologist in South Africa I have investigated many thousands of deaths, many of which were bizarre yet fascinating. Some cases are, indeed, stranger than fiction.

In this book, I will share a variety of case studies that describe a few unique experiences and particular challenges faced by forensic pathologists on the African continent. This book is about my personal journey as a forensic pathologist in South Africa. The pathology of trauma in Africa is slightly different from that in the rest of the world. As the Latin expression goes, *ex Africa semper aliquid novi* – always something new out of Africa.

For starters, the conditions under which we work are quite different from those in developed countries. In South Africa and elsewhere on the continent, forensics is often practised in a resource-depleted or resource-limited environment, the fancy-schmansy equipment like one sees on hit television series such as *CSI* simply is not available, there are regular labour relations issues such as strikes, there is often no electricity, running water or insect spray, and there are flies. Lots and lots of flies. Consequently, each day is about the small victories.

Deaths such as necklacing (when a rubber tyre is placed around the upper body and set alight), Temik (aldicarb) poisoning and deaths related to the use of traditional medicines are also specific to South Africa.

Then there is the African wildlife to contend with. Forensic pathologists see deaths from lions, leopards, buffaloes, crocodiles and the like. Furthermore, thunderstorms are a regular occurrence on the African continent; so, we see a host of lightning deaths.

South Africa even has its very own type of transport-related deaths, with cars hitting anything from donkeys to hippopotami.

Practising forensic pathology in Africa is not all doom and gloom, though. There are success stories. There are good deeds, and there are unsung heroes.

People in Africa are probably among the most resilient on earth.

To become a forensic pathologist in South Africa, you need a basic medical degree (five or six years of study), and then you need to complete two years' internship and a year of community service. Finally, you specialise, which takes another four years – assuming, obviously, that you managed to be accepted into the course, which is highly competitive. The course itself is disciplined and unrelenting, designed to weed out the weak.

Expect a life of constant exposure to death, and of sleep deprivation and long hours of practice. Generally speaking, forensic pathologists are perfectionists and high achievers. You need to keep abreast of the latest knowledge and technology. For this reason, I have been studying for over twenty-three years. For me, it has also been a life of never-ending exams and study. You constantly need to adapt to a succession of scientific, technological and sociocultural changes.

As a forensic pathologist, you should not be afraid to challenge conventional wisdom. You must endeavour to become a truly critical thinker, a sceptical enquirer and, more specifically, a medical detective. Forensic pathologists are detectives in white coats.

The consequences of resting on your reputation, stale knowledge and outdated experience can be dire. Criminals are always trying to outsmart and outwit the law. For this reason, you need to be aware of what is happening on the streets, so to speak.

You also need the mental stamina for regular exposure to death and misfortune. Forensic pathologists are exposed to disfigured and traumatically mutilated bodies on a regular basis. There are the multiple stabbing deaths, the victims of a brutal mob assault, the child abuse cases, the deaths by multiple shootings and the severely decomposed bodies, to name but a few. On average, a forensic pathologist in South Africa may end up performing, directly or indirectly, between 10 000 and 20 000 autopsies during his or her career.

Occasionally, you also have to deal with what is known as a 'hot potato' case. This is a case that is so politically charged and highly publicised that no one wants to deal with it. You may even be asked to investigate war crimes, high-profile assassinations, mass disasters and armed conflicts. For these cases, you need a really thick skin.

Very few people know what a forensic pathologist does on a day-to-day basis. In this book, I try to offer a peek behind the mysterious curtain that is forensic pathology in South Africa. These stories were gleaned from the trenches, amidst the blood and the guts of it all. I offer stories from my life and my 'case book'. When I use the word 'case', please understand that it represents a real human being who died under tragic circumstances. These were real patients who were frightened, and who suffered. Each story will be treated with the care, dignity and respect it deserves.

The Irish-Canadian politician Thomas D'Arcy McGee once said, 'We speak for the dead to protect the living.' In this book, however, I will not be speaking for the dead, but only for myself. I will be sharing my personal observations and insights based on all the deaths with which I have dealt. I will also try to answer some of the questions that members of the public have asked me most often.

No names or vital details will be mentioned in this book. Since most of the forensic pathology cases are simply too sensitive to discuss and others are *sub judice*, each case has been de-identified as much as possible.

I embarked upon this project with one simple question: What can the dead teach us, the living? I think forensic pathologists represent the final safety net in the whole of medicine. When a medicolegal question arises that no one else can seem to answer, give it to us.

Forensic pathologists have to educate up and educate down, because even people at the highest levels of government do not fully understand and appreciate what we do on a day-to-day basis.

Being constantly exposed to death and dying may be somewhat negative. However, this book will focus on the good. I have always tried my best to do the right thing; I hope that the undiluted humanity of it all will leave you feeling more positive and optimistic about life.

AUTHOR'S NOTE

Throughout this book, where the pronoun 'he' is used, it is intended that the word 'she' is equally applicable, unless obviously inappropriate from the context. Indeed, there are more female forensic pathologists practising in Southern Africa than male ones.

1

So you want to be a forensic pathologist?

'Oh my word, you're a forensic pathologist? Like in *CSI*? That must be *so* interesting! But don't you get depressed?'

This is a typical reaction I get when someone meets me for the first time and finds out what I do. I never know how best to respond. Do I try to romanticise my job and play to their fantasies? Or do I tell them the cold, hard truth?

The questions do not stop there. People usually hang around at the cocktail party or the braai, wanting *all* the curious details. The first question people usually ask is, 'What is the most interesting thing you have seen?'

At this point I stop them and say, 'I do not find other people's unnatural deaths interesting!' After all, each of the unnatural deaths I deal with represents a tragedy in someone's life. However, if you were to ask me what the most unusual or strangest thing is that I have seen, I would probably tell you the story of the giant rat.

One day, a body arrived at the mortuary. It was sealed in a metal coffin, which in turn was placed in a wooden coffin, fastened shut with steel screws. The inside of the metal coffin was filled with 100 per cent formalin.

This was quite typical: when bodies from any of the central

African countries are referred to us for a forensic autopsy examination, they are never placed in 10 per cent formalin as per best-practice occupational health and safety guidelines. Nope – it is almost always 100 per cent formalin, which means that, should you open the metal coffin indoors, you'd get very sick or die from asphyxia: the formalin would volatilise and turn the space into a gas chamber.

So, we took the coffin outdoors, removed the metal screws and poured the formalin into large metal drums for formal waste disposal. We then rinsed the contaminated body with a hosepipe.

The next moment we noticed a piece of 'wire' protruding from the region of the xiphisternum, the area below the chest plate. The deceased, a South African, had died in a plane crash in central Africa. At first, we thought the 'wire' could be part of the plane wreckage. But you can never be too safe, so we immediately had the body X-rayed. After all, it could also have been part of a bomb. Certain nefarious groups have been known to place bombs inside dead bodies to injure and even kill health professionals.

What we found was most extraordinary. It was not a bomb – it was the decomposing body of a giant rat, trapped in foetal position inside the thorax of the deceased! The rat was almost the size of the greater cane rat, which lives in reedbeds and on riverbanks in sub-Saharan Africa. Heaven knows what it was doing in the dead body.

During the embalming process, the mammal must have entered the thorax during post-mortem predation and was most likely enclosed in the thoracic cavity by post-mortem swelling of the body. Only the rat's tail – which looked exactly like a piece of wire – protruded from the body.

Other questions I am regularly asked include, What is the worst thing you have seen? The worst smell? What constitutes a good death . . . and a bad death? I am also asked, What information can be gleaned from someone's medicine cabinet? (Quite a lot.) What is the perfect murder? How can we prevent suicide? People also ask me to tell them about prison, because I also have to attend deaths in custody.

In this book I will try to answer these, and many other, questions. Take, for example, the average medicine cabinet. It will show you what medication someone is taking and if they suffer from any serious diseases, whether they use mouthwash and even if they floss regularly. Should you discover hundreds of vitamin supplements and/or omega oils, the medicine cabinet could also tell you whether someone is a hypochondriac.

The antiretroviral tablets used to help manage HIV/Aids will also generally be kept in the medicine cabinet. I once went to a scene of a dyadic death (a murder–suicide). The husband had shot and killed his wife, and then himself. Examination of the open medicine cabinet showed a container of antiretroviral drugs; some were also present on a nearby table. My theory is that either the husband did not know that his wife was on antiretrovirals and found out when he saw the pills, or he knew they both had HIV/Aids and may have killed his wife and himself for this reason. Sadly, the answer will never be known.

Most of the suicide and dyadic death cases I have seen had a background history of HIV/Aids. This, I believe, is due to poor initial counselling. If only people knew and understood that HIV/Aids can be treated like any other chronic natural disease (such as hypertension and diabetes mellitus). Most people die *with* their HIV and not *because* of it. This was a really tragic case. Of course, my theories are merely speculation. Most other cases of dyadic deaths were shown to be due to love triangles.

Another question I'm frequently asked is, What is the quickest and the most painless way to die? I usually answer by saying, Please try to focus on life. But to answer this somewhat morbid question: personally, I would like to die in the arms of a woman, slightly drunk, slightly in love and due to a massive myocardial infarction. That should be a relatively quick and painless death.

Failing that, I think a nuclear death, or a lightning death, or jumping into an active volcano would probably be the quickest death to endure. Another swift way to die would be assassination by a sniper. Not just any sniper, but a really good sniper with a really good rifle and a high-velocity, large-calibre projectile, from behind the head. On a balance of probabilities, this would probably be the ultimate way to go.

Paradoxically, a guillotine or a gunshot wound through the temples of the head with a low-velocity weapon would be a relatively slow death in comparison. With a guillotine, for example, the blood might pump through the vessels in your neck at about 70 ml of blood per pump for the next thirty or so minutes. Unless the projectile goes through the brainstem, it won't be a rapid death. (There is a cubic centimetre of brain tissue in the brainstem where your vasomotor and cardiorespiratory centres are located.) Aiming for the brainstem would ensure a relatively quick and painless death – you would drop to the ground like a sack of potatoes.

There are many cases of botched suicides where people who tried to shoot themselves through the temples merely took out their eyes and went blind. There are also cases where people who shot themselves through the roof of the mouth and out the frontal lobes of the brain have opened the front door for the paramedics. Then, I know of an individual who had been stabbed in the heart yet managed to kill someone before finally succumbing to his heart injury.

On the flip side, in certain cultures in South Africa people actually wish for a slow, drawn-out death, since they want to have time to say goodbye to all their loved ones and friends before they die.

What is death? Death is an unavoidable change which occurs in everybody's life. It is feared by many, but welcomed by others. If you are terminally ill, you may welcome death. If you are young and mighty, death is a foe.[1] Death has also been described as one of man's greatest and most exciting experiences.[2]

Death and the process of dying are characterised by loss of function of the great organ systems (the cardiovascular, respiratory and nervous systems) and their coordination. This reveals a dissociation of the function of the different organs. The agonal period may be initiated either by disease or by trauma. The period of dying is called 'agony' and its duration can vary depending on the damaging agent and the remaining facilities of the patient.

The final crisis leads to a state of *vita minima* (state of apparent death) in which no vital signs are apparent, and to a state of death characterised by irreversible cessation of circulation or by respiratory arrest. Under special clinical conditions, brain death may replace the classic signs of death – that is, irreversible circulatory or respiratory arrest and its consequences.[3]

The medical practitioner in general practice, or a specialist, is expected to establish whether death has occurred or not. At times, the diagnosis of death may be extremely difficult; often, even the most experienced practitioners are fooled because so-called death mimics can occur.

Once, an elderly woman whose normal bodily functions had apparently ceased was admitted to the hospital at which I was working. I could hardly hear her heartbeat, there was no respiration and her temperature was hypothermic – that is, well below normal. Fearing the worst, I immediately covered her with a space blanket, gave her oxygen and inserted an intravenous line in a collapsed vein in her arm. I went to speak to her family and told them that I did not expect their granny to survive for much longer. To my very great surprise, when I returned to her ward she was sitting up, listening to the radio and eating crisps! Hypothermia is a very good death mimic, and I was badly fooled.

There are many ways to die, but it is important to distinguish between natural and unnatural deaths. Depending on which agencies' data you review, South Africa has between 300 000 and 600 000 natural deaths per year, with an average of approximately 500 000 per year. These encompass deaths from heart attacks to strokes to cancer, for example. Those who die in this way will generally not undergo a forensic autopsy but may undergo a hospital autopsy performed by an anatomical pathologist, especially where the death is due to natural causes but the natural disease is unknown. The deceased's family would have to consent to an anatomical pathology autopsy.

Forensic pathologists perform autopsies on unnatural deaths only. Altogether, there are approximately 60 000 to 80 000 unnatural deaths per year in South Africa, with an average of 70 000 per year. An unnatural death may be defined as:

- a death caused by the application of a force or any other physical or chemical factor, direct or indirect, and with or without complications
- any death which, in the medical practitioner's opinion, was caused by an act or an omission on somebody's part
- a death in terms of section 56 of the Health Professions Act (Act 56 of 1974), which states that '[t]he death of a person whilst under the influence of a general anaesthetic or local anaesthetic, or of which the administration of an anaesthetic has been a contributory cause, shall not be deemed to be a death from natural causes', these are also known as procedure-related or procedure-associated deaths
- any unattended, unexplained, suspicious or sudden unexpected death.

The medicolegal investigation of death in South Africa has a very strict legislative framework. The field is highly regulated; many Acts legislate it, such as the Inquests Act (Act 58 of 1959); the Registration of Births and Deaths Act (Act 51 of 1992); the National Health Act (Act 61 of 2003); the Health Professions Act (Act 56 of 1974); and the Criminal Procedure Act (Act 51 of 1977). There is also the National Code of Guidelines for Forensic Pathology Practice in South Africa, and the Rules and Regulations of the Health Professions Council of South Africa.

Sadly, next of kin may not refuse a medicolegal autopsy. The State has absolute authority in this regard. If someone dies an unnatural death in South Africa, a full medicolegal inquest will be required. Forensic pathologists help conduct the medicolegal investigation, which includes an investigation of the circumstances surrounding the death. The autopsy is but one small component of the death investigation. Forensic pathologists are therefore specialist death investigators who help bring closure. We are here to serve, to solve and to soothe.

To the layperson, it would seem that forensic pathologists must know almost everything there is to know about death. Which is true, in part. However, what laypeople do not really know is that forensic pathologists chiefly deal with no more than about twenty-four ways of unnatural death. We must know everything about these twenty-four forensic topics.

The main forensic topics are deaths related to sharp force trauma, blunt force trauma, transportation, gunshots and explosions, burns and scalds, abuses of human rights, electrical fatalities, suffocation and asphyxia, fatal pressure on the neck, immersion deaths, neglect, starvation and hypothermia, deaths associated with sexual offences, certain pregnancy-related deaths, child deaths, surgical procedures, dysbaric and barotrauma-related deaths (deaths due to sudden changes in atmospheric pressure), and the pathology of sudden death and poisoning.

Forensic pathologists help determine the cause and manner of death; help to identify the deceased, if his or her identity is unknown; determine the time of death and injury; collect evidence; document injuries or the lack of them; help deduce how the injuries occurred; document any underlying natural disease present; attend the scene of death; determine or exclude other contributory factors; and provide expert testimony if a case goes to trial.[4]

Often, huge amounts of money are at stake, depending on whether a death resulted from injury at work, whether a shooting was accidental or suicidal, or whether a heart attack occurred before, during, or after a motor vehicle accident.

Forensic pathologists also take part in exercises in preventative medicine – which is part of the purpose of this book. Forewarned is forearmed!

In my opinion, no other field in medicine offers the intellectual challenge of forensic pathology, as it requires a working knowledge of diagnosis and treatment in almost every speciality of medicine. It is probably the most integrative branch of medicine. It calls for an understanding of non-medical fields like criminology, criminalistics, engineering, highway design, forensic science and a deep understanding of the community – its mores, folkways and religion. For this reason, one can say that a forensic pathologist conducts a medicolegal examination like a conductor does an orchestra.

Although there are differences among countries, the philosophy behind forensic pathology has always remained the same: 'The application of medical knowledge and methodology for the resolution of legal questions and problems for individuals and societies.'[5] As mentioned earlier, without good legal medicine, there can never be good justice.

Forensic *medicine* may be defined as consisting essentially of that body of medical and paramedical scientific knowledge that may be used for the purposes of administration of the law.[6] The basic mission of forensic medicine is the proper application of justice.[7] Much of what justice has been in the past few centuries has passed through forensic medicine, and much of what justice ought to be will pass through it in the future.

Forensic *science*, on the other hand, refers to the actual examination of scenes of death, recovery of evidence, laboratory examinations, and interpretation of findings and presentation of the conclusions for use in court. Activities range from instrumental analysis, such as analysis of blood alcohol and drugs, to DNA typing of items at the scene of a crime.

When I first meet someone, my eyes immediately wander to the 'forensically significant' aspects of their body and their behaviour. I check their skin. Do they have tattoos? I check the condition of their teeth. I look at their posture and the clothes they are wearing. Is one hand slightly paler than their other hand? I notice their perfume and/or aftershave. I even check their nails.

This happens within milliseconds – even before I have made eye contact. By the time I greet them, I already have an image, in my forensic mind's eye, of their general health, their mindset and the risks they take.

I have always been fascinated by the undiscovered and the undiscoverable. It was a combination of the stories of Dr Joseph Bell and Sir Arthur Conan Doyle that inspired me to become a forensic pathologist. Conan Doyle's *The Sign of Four* (1890) opens with a scene in which Dr Watson hands a recently inherited pocket watch to his friend Sherlock Holmes and challenges him to describe the character of its late owner.

After a brief examination of the watch, Holmes comments that presumably it belonged to Watson's elder brother. Watson says that Holmes is right in this, but points out that he could have guessed it from the initials on the watch case. Amused at his friend's seeming failure, Watson asks if Holmes has any other deductions: 'He was a man of untidy habits – very untidy and careless. He was left with good prospects, but he threw away his chances, lived for some time in poverty with occasional short intervals of prosperity, and, finally, taking to drink, he died. That is all I can gather.'

As to how Holmes did it, you'll have to read the book – which is brilliant, I might add.

Holmes calls this the facility of 'reasoning backwards'. First, you must learn to notice things, to become aware of every possible detail – and second, you must be able to analyse what you see to determine which action or situation brought it about.

To quote Holmes: 'Let the enquirer begin by . . . on meeting a fellow mortal, learning at a glance to distinguish the history of the man, and the trade or profession to which he belongs . . . by a man's finger-nails, by his coat-sleeve, by his boots, by his trouser-knees, by the callosities of his forefinger and thumb, by his expression, by his shirt-cuff – by each of these things a man's calling is plainly revealed.'[8]

This technique of reasoning backwards is difficult to teach, although it is not impossible to learn. Both the dead and the living have a lot to teach us. I once predicted a woman's divorce based on her sudden and dramatic change in hairstyle, and I know from experience that many suicides of middle-aged women are preceded by this change.

A woman's hairstyle is one of her most important physical attributes. A major change may point to some unresolved internal psychological conflict. One such a case involved a woman who had complained bitterly about her unfulfilling marriage and filed for divorce. She was found dead after drinking a 'milkshake' of crushed, mixed drugs. Shortly before that, she had dramatically changed her hairstyle. For this reason, my advice to men is to take very careful note of their wife's or partner's hairstyle.

Or take the following example where I learnt so much just by casual observation after meeting a woman in the queue at a shop. Her lips looked like they were recovering from beestings (she had had Botox injections) and her skin had lost its natural lustre (she was a smoker). From the brands of the clothing she was wearing, I could deduce that she was within a certain income bracket. Her posture and her weight gave me an idea of whether she did any exercise and allowed me a relatively good guess at her dietary habits. I also noticed multiple parallel incision scars on the wrist of her less dominant hand, which told me she had had previous suicide attempts.

These kinds of subtle insights you won't find in any of the mainstream textbooks. They pertain to undiscovered aspects of human behaviour of which the average person seems to be blissfully unaware. You obtain this knowledge from being fortunate enough to find yourself in the right place and in the right job – in the mortuary, as a forensic pathologist. Or, as I call it, in the blind spot of humanity.

2

My last living patient

Before I became a forensic pathologist, I practised as a general practitioner. I did my internship in Cape Town at Somerset Hospital and my community service in Phalaborwa at a small rural hospital called Maphutha Malatji Hospital. A few critical incidents over this period helped me decide to become a forensic pathologist.

The first incident occurred in February 2012, when tropical cyclone Leon-Eline brought gusty winds and torrential rain to Madagascar, Mozambique and the northeastern parts of Southern Africa. Eline is still considered one of the most devastating tropical cyclones of the 2011–2012 season.

That night, I was called to Maphutha Malatji because a heavily pregnant woman was experiencing foetal distress. It was raining heavily. I assessed the woman and ascertained that she needed an emergency caesarean section. I phoned my second on call, who still had to drive from his home to the hospital.

The woman was in severe pain and the foetal distress was escalating. When my second on call still hadn't arrived after a while, I called again. He told me that there was no way he was going to be able to reach the hospital: the rivers had flooded. I was on my own.

That was the night Irina made landfall. I ended up being trapped in that 200-bed hospital for two days and two nights before the rivers finally subsided and it was safe for me to drive back to town. I was the only doctor in the hospital. It was me and a handful of nursing sisters.

That night, I performed the caesarean section alone with two nursing sisters. I had to perform the anaesthetic and operation by myself. In the middle of the procedure, the power went off and we had to work under the light of a laryngoscope blade and candles. I am happy to report that both the mother and the baby survived.

Those two days and two nights are a bit of a blur to me. I had to practise what can only be described as wilderness medicine, which means doing what you can with what you have at the time. I had minimal sleep over those two days. Needless to say, it was a surreal and stressful time, but I learnt a lot about myself. For one thing, the self-reliance it taught me was invaluable. There was no one to help me and no expert to whom I could turn for advice. I simply had to make a plan under the flickering light of those candles. As I reflect on these events, I can still recall the depth of my fear and my anxiety.

Over those two days, many people came into the hospital with fractures from the tropical storm. Interestingly, those who lived in traditional mud-and-thatch huts had fewer injuries than those who lived in makeshift corrugated-iron shacks. This suggested to me that our ancestors probably had greater wisdom than us moderns.

Tropical Storm Irina also gave me my first taste of dealing with mass casualties. Mass disasters have different definitions, but the generally accepted definition is an event that overwhelms local resources. Mass disasters are fortunately relatively rare events, but when they do occur they tend to place excessive strain on medical services. Today, mass disaster management is a speciality in forensic pathology.

It was during my time in Phalaborwa that I attended my first autopsy. A miner, who had worked in one of the many mines around the town, had died unexpectedly. A private forensic pathologist had been consulted and flown up from one of the big cities to perform the autopsy.

I attended in a watching brief capacity. All I knew about forensic pathology at the time was from the 1976 American hit television series *Quincy, M.E.*, which was about a county medical examiner who investigated clues about what appeared to be suspicious deaths. Suddenly, I had the opportunity to witness a real-life autopsy in person; I jumped at it.

At first, the autopsy overwhelmed my senses. I did not know what I was seeing; it all just looked like one bloody mess. It was a completely disorientating sensory experience. I can still recall the sights, sounds and smells. At the time, I also had no idea of what was 'normal' and what was 'abnormal' during an autopsy. I couldn't see the difference between normal injuries that had occurred while the miner was still alive and injuries that were caused after his death by the dissection of the body and organs.

I was intrigued, encouraged and a little bit overwhelmed. It was unlike anything I had ever witnessed before. Like most youngsters, I had been brainwashed into thinking that you became a medical doctor to save the living. My first autopsy experience made me wonder if this was indeed true.

Becoming a pathologist was not something I had even considered before. Luckily, I had a good guide – you need such a guide, someone who has walked and hacked open the path before you.

There were many perspectives surrounding the sudden, unexpected death of the miner that piqued my curiosity. For one, it transpired that the miner had been murdered. His co-workers suspected that he had died from hyperthermia, but in fact the cause of death was blunt force trauma to the head.

I am often asked what is considered normal and what is considered pathology. I usually try to explain the concept of pathology to laypeople as follows: How does an expert game ranger spot a leopard in the African bush? The answer is: with expert knowledge based on experience.

If the game ranger drives a particular stretch of bush every day, he will know that stretch of bush like the back of his hand. Every day, he will see the same rocky outcrop. One day, the outline of the outcrop will look slightly different. His 'diagnosis'? A leopard is lying on the rocky outcrop.

The game ranger knows what is 'normal', and will therefore be able to spot when something is out of the ordinary, or 'abnormal'. So too in pathology and forensic pathology. To 'spot' pathology in the heart, for example, you first need to know what constitutes a normal heart.

Before you enter the field of forensic pathology, you have to interrogate your motives thoroughly. It might sound cool to be a forensic pathologist, but what keeps you going after the 9 000th autopsy? What keeps you motivated? I often compare it to running an ultramarathon. What would compel you to participate? Is it your ego or a greater calling?

I got into this field firstly because I could not tolerate injustice and secondly because I wanted to help real victims. What do I mean by 'real' victims, you may ask? Let me tell you a story from the time shortly after I had completed my community service in rural Limpopo.

In 2001, I left for the United Kingdom to do a year's clinical medicine. Soon, I found myself practising medicine at St Luke's Hospital and Bradford Royal Infirmary. I worked in the emergency medicine department and did a stint in the discipline of geriatric medicine. I also spent about six months taking care of accidents and emergencies in that part of the world.

One night, I was already asleep when I got a call from the emergency room. It was about 3 a.m. on a bitterly cold night; I recall having had to put on several layers of clothing and a jacket and trudge across a courtyard covered in knee-deep snow.

Waiting for me was an elderly white male who presented with an acute asthma attack. He was near extremis – very close to dying. The entire emergency room team worked to bring him back to normality, with much energy, stress and medication.

After the drama had subsided, I asked the elderly gentleman whether he smoked.

'Fifty fags a day, lad! Fifty fags a day!' was his somewhat arrogant response.

I leaned forward, and mentioned that he was wasting all of our time. I may have used an expletive between 'our' and 'time', although the specific details of that conversation elude me.

One of the nursing sisters rushed up and started scolding me. 'We do not talk to our patients like that!'

'This guy has disrupted our entire night because he continues to smoke like a chimney! Why can't I reprimand him?'

'Patients will do whatever they want to do. It is a free world. He is well within his rights to smoke!' the nursing sister barked at me.

I did not sign up for this, I thought. I went into medicine to help innocent victims, but this guy was here because of bad personal choices. I was in no mood to discuss the principle of luck egalitarianism with the nursing sister at 4 a.m. – that sometimes bad things happen to good people through no fault of their own, and at other times because of their own bad choices.

'This is not right,' I said. When the shift ended, I handed in my resignation and quit clinical medicine.

The realisation hit me like a ton of bricks: like most health professionals, I went into medicine to try to help people. Yet the ill were not always that innocent and many were beyond help. Many ate too much, drank unhealthy drinks, had un-protected sex, drove fast cars without wearing seatbelts and popped multiple pills. Others smoked or watched television all day without caring about their health.

In medicine, acute conditions are treated acutely and chronic conditions are treated chronically. In other words, if it happens quickly (such as a fractured ankle), you treat it quickly. If it develops slowly over years (high blood pressure, diabetes from bad diet, etc.), the treatment will most likely take years. It always irked me in clinical practice how the morbidly obese person wanted to be treated *now*.

I felt morally injured by all of this and decided, there and then, that my energy, talents, skills and knowledge would be better spent helping real victims. I felt like I was wasting my time trying to save people as a general practitioner. It was then that I enrolled in forensic pathology. Luckily, I got accepted at a prestigious university that admitted only two registrars every four years.

To become a forensic pathologist, you must either become an anatomical pathologist first and then super specialise in forensic pathology, or complete a forensic pathology degree. This depends on where you wish to specialise, because some countries do not have such a degree. Fortunately, South Africa does offer it and it is highly sought after, both nationally and internationally.

Upon completion of your academic degree, additional training is required. Internationally, the average study time from entering university to becoming a fully qualified and practising forensic pathologist is approximately fourteen years. Obviously, there are differences in different countries as to how you become a board-certified forensic pathologist.

In South Africa's more rural areas, autopsies are mostly performed by general practitioners. Some of the general practitioners have a diploma in forensic medicine, which could take up to three years to obtain. Full-time forensic pathologists like me tend to work in large cities, primarily because a reasonably large population base is required to support a full-time forensic pathologist. A hardworking forensic pathologist could investigate up to 500 cases per year. At the time of writing, South Africa had 53 to 56 qualified full-time forensic pathologists for a population of approximately 57.4 million.

Suffice to say that one gets a spectrum of autopsies in South Africa. Depending on the facility and the qualifications of the forensic pathologist or general practitioner involved, the quality of the autopsy may range from 'gourmet' to 'peekaboo'.

Some autopsies are excellent; others are very poor indeed. Well-functioning death investigation systems are headed by forensic pathologists who retain the power to investigate deaths of community concern. In fact, forensic pathology might well be called community and public safety pathology.

My days as a forensic pathologist are certainly varied. One day I might be stuck behind my microscope, where the world seems so small. On another day I might find myself on top of a high mountain or deep in a cave or at the scene of a mass disaster, and the world seems so big.

However, most of the time I am in my autopsy suite conducting post-mortems. Forensic pathologists tend to work quietly in the mortuary, which is typically found in the basement of some or other hospital or behind some or other police station. The international trend nowadays, however, is to build more modern, state-of-the-art mortuaries with abundant natural light and open space. The idea is to take forensic pathology out of the basement.

You may not believe it, but some of the mortuaries in South Africa are of the most beautiful in the world. The gardens will truly astound you. There are comfort gardens designed to attract birds and butterflies. There are designated areas for forensically significant plants, which serve as educational tools for students and visitors. Certain mortuaries have flowing water features, fountains and indigenous trees, to help comfort the bereaved.

Even though we deal chiefly with the dead, we also deal with the living: police, detectives, paramedics, medical students, prosecutors, lawyers, judges, criminals and members of the public. The forensic pathologist is just one link in a long chain of investigators. On a single investigation you may find not only police detectives but also ballistics experts, forensic photographers, crime scene reconstruction experts, DNA experts, forensic anthropologists, forensic entomologists, forensic odontologists, forensic cybercrime experts, etc.

Forensic pathology can be a thankless job. We arrive at work early and we only get home late. Often, we work under extremely challenging conditions. In winter, the mortuary can be freezing cold, often colder than it is outdoors. And in summer, the mortuary can be extremely hot on days when the air conditioners are not working, often hotter than it is outdoors.

Furthermore, forensic pathology is about as well paid as the clergy, only with much longer working hours and no promise of eternal salvation at the end! Salaries pale in comparison to those of other medical specialities, yet we need the same level of understanding as the other specialities. For example, if someone dies on the operating table while undergoing a Nissen fundoplication (a surgical procedure to treat gastroesophageal reflux disease or hiatal hernia), the forensic pathologist will have to know almost everything there is to know about Nissen fundoplications. So too with craniotomies, cardiac surgery, bladder surgery, spinal surgery, etc. Forensic pathologists have to understand anaesthesia and anaesthetic drugs. Yet we earn a fraction of the money that these other specialities earn.

Regarding funding, forensic pathology is always going to come last on the list because our patients are already dead. The money in medicine chiefly goes to maternal health, child health, tuberculosis and HIV/Aids.

In the *American Journal of Forensic Medicine and Pathology*, Ronald Wright and Larry Tate write: 'The forensic pathologist finds himself making "house calls" in the wee hours of the morning, testifying in court, studying electrical theory or consoling the family of a baby who has died from sudden infant death syndrome. He may be doing research on the correlation of injuries with vehicle design or the effect and effectiveness of out-of-hospital cardiopulmonary resuscitation. No matter what activities man may be involved in, things will go wrong, deaths will result, and the forensic pathologist will be expected to answer why and what might be done to prevent needless deaths.'[9]

So, what motivates me? What keeps me going after the 9 000th autopsy?

It's my personal fight against injustice, which was awakened many years ago when I was in high school. The day before my final high school examinations, my suitcase with all my books in it was stolen. I was a mega-nerd and I coveted my textbooks. If I'd got bad marks for my final exams, I would never have got into medicine. I managed to solve the mystery of my missing school suitcase, but it took me three hours of extreme stress to find and confront the guilty parties. They confessed to having hidden it as a joke.

Injustice boils my blood. How can people be so cruel? I understood at a very young age that there are people who are wired completely differently from me. I realised that there are people who want to maintain peace, and there are people who want to disrupt it. Some people wake up in the morning with the desire to harm others; they will steal from little old grannies and even commit murder.

Even when you look at bone tissue under the microscope, you'll find osteoblasts and osteoclasts. An osteoblast is a cell that secretes the substance of bone; an osteoclast is a large multinucleate bone cell that absorbs bone tissue during growth and healing. The one cell builds bone; the other cell destroys it. Even at a cellular level, creation and destruction seem to co-exist.

I have been the victim of injustice several times in my own life. I, too, have been the victim of crime. Today, the helplessness I have felt as a victim is my fuel. Part of me wants to be a superhero who goes on a vigilante revenge spree, hunting down the bad guys. Sadly, nerd that I am, I will probably end up on my own dissection table before the bad guys do.

I realised that my only resource was my brain and my mind. I wanted to put the bad guys behind bars legally, using logic and science as my weapon. Laws, sadly, don't stop evil men. Good men stop evil men. Since then, my entire life's work has been dedicated to learning, medicine and forensics. Forensics is in my DNA.

Knowing that I am addressing injustice is what keeps me motivated. The intangible thrill of catching bad guys is what drives me. Solving puzzles is what makes me get up in the morning and keeps me going.

3

Autopsies and exhumations

When I was a youngster, I loved watching *Quincy, M.E.*, starring Jack Klugman as a Los Angeles County medical examiner. The introductory scenes to *Quincy* show a medical student fainting as Quincy dramatically whips away a blanket, exposing a corpse. I suspect quite a few people might have such a scene in mind when they think of an autopsy.

The autopsy is centuries old and the skills surrounding it have been honed over hundreds of years. Even in the most primitive tribal societies there was an interest in discovering causes of death. In particular, an unexpected or unwitnessed death could have signalled a potential danger, from within the society or from an outside enemy.

As societies started to develop and became more organised, also in terms of their judicial systems, the forensic investigation of deaths was introduced. The oldest known official instructions about the external investigation of corpses have been dated to ancient China.

One of the first books about post-mortem examinations – *Xi Yuan Ji Lu* [The Washing Away of Wrongs] – was written in Chinese by Song Ci and published in 1247. Song Ci wrote that a forensic medical doctor must be serious, conscientious

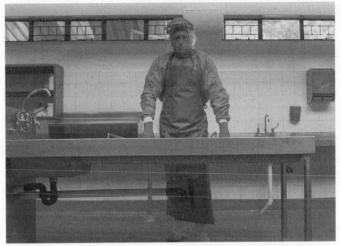

Some of the personal protective equipment required to perform a medicolegal autopsy. *Photo: E de Pauw and D Fisher (Walla Films)*

and highly responsible, and must also personally examine each dead body or that of a wounded person. The particulars of each case must be recorded in the doctor's own handwriting. No one else is allowed to write his autopsy report.

He must not avoid performing an autopsy because he detests the stench of corpses. He must refrain from sitting comfortably behind a curtain of incense that masks the stench, let his subordinates do the autopsy unsupervised, or allow a petty official to write his autopsy report, leaving all the inaccuracies unchecked and uncorrected.

The earliest known forensic dissections took place in Italy in the middle of the thirteenth century. Over the course of the centuries that followed, autopsies were increasingly performed and recorded, contributing to the advancement of pathology and, of course, mankind.

The medicolegal or forensic autopsy is performed on the

instructions of the legal authority responsible for the investigation of sudden, suspicious, obscure, unnatural, litigious, unexplained, questionable or criminal deaths. In most judicial systems, permission for medicolegal autopsy from the relatives of the deceased is not required. After all, the murderer may be one of the relatives of the deceased. For this reason, autopsies are performed on the authority of the state. Although there are differences between countries, this philosophy has always remained the same.

To the forensic pathologist, a corpse represents a crime scene that potentially contains many clues about the cause of death. The autopsy is a way to uncover these clues. It is a very complex and labour-intensive procedure, but also one of the cheapest procedures in medicine. An autopsy is also the biggest procedure in the whole of medicine (never let a surgeon tell you otherwise!).

What are the tools of the trade for a forensic pathologist? Firstly, you need personal protective equipment like gloves, gowns, aprons, masks, goggles or a visor mask and Wellington-like boots. Personal protective equipment is now a super speciality in and of itself. Metal and synthetic mesh gloves worn underneath surgical gloves can mitigate the risk of autopsy injuries from scalpels and other sharp objects, but they offer no protection from needle punctures, for example.

Then, you require a scalpel, forceps, a few long knives, an oscillating head saw to remove the skull bone (if this saw is broken, or unavailable, a normal hacksaw should suffice), pincers, scissors, a measuring jug, a scale, sponges, a good autopsy table, a decent working surface, down-draft air conditioners, a good, solid floor, a good drainage system, good light and – most importantly – running water.

We need sharp knives and scissors to cut, a pincer or forceps to grasp, and a ruler to measure the dimensions of wounds or tumours. The measuring jug is to measure collections of fluid, pus or blood, and we need sponges to clean and a scale to weigh organs. We need body bags, evidence and specimen collection containers, toe tags and an adequate labelling system for specimens.

Reconstruction of the body after post-mortem examination is also a vital part of the autopsy. Preservation of the dignity of the deceased remains our highest priority. Necessity dictates absolute care and respect for the dead. All the organs are carefully replaced in the body after autopsy. All wounds are cosmetically closed and reconstructed. Even in cases such as mutilation or beheadings, the body must be reconstructed, cleaned and presented back to the family or loved ones for cremation or burial.

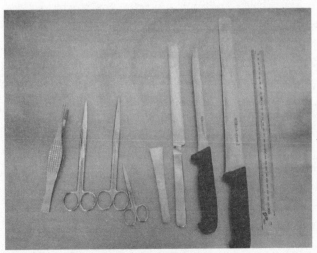

Forceps, different scissors and knives, and a ruler are some of the tools used by a forensic pathologist. *Photo: R Blumenthal*

There are perhaps a handful of post-mortem cosmetic experts practising in South Africa. Sadly, no such course is offered locally. These experts have typically studied abroad and have the knowledge to preserve and reconstruct bodies for viewing purposes. They may inject certain dyes and perfumes into the veins of the deceased and have the skills to make jaundiced or anaemic patients look almost normal. Some of these experts even suture wounds with the same skill as a plastic surgeon.

Everything else – including X-ray machines, CT machines, MRI machines, and biochemistry and toxicology laboratories – is considered a luxury when practising forensics in a resource-limited or resource-depleted environment. Sometimes, the physical plant in which we work is not robust enough for this kind of work. I have seen colleagues from other African countries perform autopsies in very poor facilities, their boots and socks drenched in their own sweat.

You would be surprised by what can be diagnosed with the most basic of senses: sight, hearing, touch and smell. One can practise good medicine with only the barest of necessities. The fanciest mortuaries may be staffed with poor forensic pathologists and the final autopsy reports will be poor. Alternatively, the most basic of mortuaries may be staffed with excellent forensic pathologists, and the final autopsy reports will be good.

However, there are certain must-haves. Forensic pathologists cannot function without running water, proper lighting, a good drainage system and electricity. Add to that good teamwork. Nice-to-haves are body bags, decent specimen collection containers, stationery, security, electronics such as computers and cameras, vehicles, and personal protective equipment such as headgear and proper eye protection. In the trenches, one person's must-haves are another person's nice-to-haves.

Regarding the mechanics of the autopsy itself, first a thorough external examination is performed. Everything is looked for and sought out. We really try to look everywhere on the body, including the very obscure places. In one case, I saw a needle puncture mark on the dorsal vein of the penis of an intravenous drug user.

We even look between the toes, up the nostrils and in the ears. Lightning deaths, for example, can sometimes only be diagnosed by a ruptured eardrum. I have also seen a host of foreign bodies up nostrils over the course of my career. One of the strangest nostril-related deaths I have seen involved a blesbok horn that penetrated a gamekeeper's nostril and fractured through the top of the skull.

Flies tend to lay their eggs in ears and nostrils. To the rookie pathologist, the compact white-yellow masses of fly eggs will look exactly like wads of cotton wool placed in the nostrils or external auditory canals. If you are not careful, they can fool you quite badly.

One should also examine the body under different light sources: white light, infrared light and ultraviolet light. Sometimes the forensically significant stuff, such as semen or dandruff, can only be seen under a specific light source. Different light sources are a luxury item in a resource-limited environment. Beware of mistaking the unobserved for the unobservable, an important topic I'll return to in a later chapter. Your not seeing it does not mean it is not there.

All the good stuff in forensic pathology tends to be on the outside of the body, whereas all the good stuff in anatomical pathology tends to be on the inside of the body. Therefore, forensic examination of the clothing is crucial.

When people wake up in the morning, they have no idea that the items they put on that day could be the last clothes they ever wear. Often, we find people dead in their home, wearing their pyjamas or only their underwear. The motor vehicle accident driver cases typically happen after a night out on the town, so the drivers and passengers are usually wearing their best outfits. Sometimes one can still smell the after-shave and perfume on the deceased.

Pedestrians are typically wearing dark-coloured clothing (which makes it difficult to see them at night). Rarely does one find a pedestrian vehicle accident case in which the victim is dressed in bright and/or neon-coloured clothing.

In winter, the bodies are covered with layer upon layer of clothing, which makes undressing them very labour intensive. We always examine people's pockets, since we need to know what people have on them at the time of death. A rookie mistake is immediately putting your gloved hand into the pocket of a deceased individual. One never knows what is inside. There may be an uncapped needle in the pocket, for example. Therefore, we have strict protocols when it comes to examining pockets. The most common item found in the pockets of deceased South Africans is a tin of Zam-Buk, a type of lip balm. We have also found used and unused condoms, drugs, weapons, Viagra, and a variety of other paraphernalia.

Sometimes, people hide things in their clothing. We have found drugs in the lining and inner seams of clothing, and money in brassieres. We have also discovered drugs and sui-cide notes in the small pockets of denim jeans. People also hide money in their socks and on their person. We have found thousands of rands over the years hidden on bodies.

I can also tell you what the most popular brand of underwear in South Africa is . . .

The brand and style of the deceased's shoes also tells us something about the person or of a crime. How someone tied their laces will tell you whether they are left- or right-handed. Once, a known murderer had washed his blood-splattered clothes, but had forgotten to clean his shoes. We found the victim's blood on the inside of one of his shoes.

Everything must be looked for on the clothing, from sand and grass scuff marks on the knee areas to missing buttons to body fluid stains. In a pedestrian vehicle accident case, the victim may have a scuff mark on the base of their shoe from being swept violently off their feet by the impact. Missing buttons may be found after physical altercations. Torn and tattered clothing is often seen in assault cases. Even the leaf debris on the clothing tells us a story. Leaf debris found on a deceased person's clothing may tell us exactly where the person was murdered.

One such case involved a deceased woman discovered on a side street. Careful examination showed leaf debris under her body from a common oak tree (*Quercus robur*) and a pecan nut tree (*Carya illinoinensis*). Yet there were no common oaks or pecan nut trees in that particular street. An investigation ensued, which included drone assessment of the neighbourhood for different types of trees. A relatively nearby property had both types of trees growing in the garden. We had found the location of the killer; the leaf debris proved pivotal in solving that case.

Lightning also tends to leave its mark on the clothing of the deceased. Torn clothing, melted fibres, ruptured shoes and torn belts are the typical signs of someone having been struck by lightning.

One of the best examples of clothing-related clues concerns the death of a young woman. Careful examination showed that her clothing seemed to have been put on by someone else. The autopsy showed that she had been raped. The rapist re-dressed his victim after killing her, but he failed to realise that he had put her belt on the wrong way. The victim had also clearly not tied her own shoelaces. What we originally suspected to be a sudden unexpected death turned out to be a rape and murder case.

I have also seen people who were killed by their own clothing. One man's tie got caught in a paper shredder and strangled him to death. There have been cases of scarves being caught in washing machine rollers and people's clothing being caught in turning or rotating factory machines.

In one case, the shirt of a man who climbed over a palisade fence got caught on one of the palisades, which left him hanging from the fence. Death was due to a complex interaction of positional asphyxia and decreased venous return. In layperson's terms: he hung in a position that compromised his normal breathing and blood flow; he slowly suffocated.

It is only after a thorough external general examination of the clothing and the body that one proceeds with the standard autopsy itself. Nowadays, bodies are thoroughly photographed and filmed before autopsy. In some forensic centres in South Africa, it is possible to perform three-dimensional surface scanning of the wounds, DNA swabbing of victims, extensive trace evidence collection, and X-ray, CT and MRI of the body. Sadly, this is the exception, not the rule.

The principles of dissection may be found in any standard autopsy textbook. Generally speaking, there will be a linear incision from below the chin to the pubic bone. A so-called Y incision, which extends from behind each ear to the jugular notch and then downwards to the pubic bone, is sometimes also made.

Organs are removed in certain 'blocks' or 'plucks'. There is the chest pluck (containing the tongue, trachea, oesophagus, heart and lungs), the abdominal pluck (containing the liver, spleen, pancreas, duodenum and stomach) and the genito-urinary pluck (containing the kidneys, ureter, bladder and internal sexual organs in the case of females). The intracranial contents are removed separately.

There are many different ways to perform an autopsy and certain special dissection techniques, such as one that looks at the posterior aspect of the neck and one to examine the heart in suspected air-embolism cases. A special technique can be used to examine the lungs if one suspects pneumothorax (air in the chest cavity), for example. We even have special techniques to look underneath the skin in certain blunt force trauma cases.

During and following a thorough autopsy examination, a multitude of special investigations may be performed, such as histology, DNA sampling, biochemical sampling, virology sampling, microbiological sampling and genetic sampling. All of these special investigations cost a lot of money. Although these investigations may be performed as routine in some

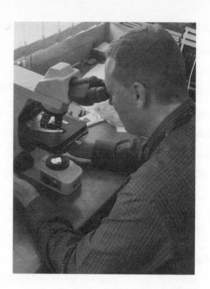

Most days are spent behind the micro-scope, where the world seems so small.

developed countries, each must be thoroughly motivated for in South Africa.

Of course, practice makes perfect, and the rookie forensic pathologist is bound to make a few mistakes during an autopsy. A common one is to mistake the normal post-mortem skin-colour change that happens over the lower right quadrant of the abdomen for a bruise. You'll often hear a rookie say, 'Hey, this guy was kicked in the stomach.' The caecum of the large intestine is found in that part of the abdomen. It fills with post-mortem gas and floats upwards towards the abdominal wall. The multiple bacteria discolour the wall, giving it the appearance of a bruise. Therefore, it is a normal skin-colour change that happens to nearly every corpse in the early stages of decomposition.

In pathology we sometimes use a huge band saw, the type with the large, spinning, serrated wheel typically seen in butcher shops. This huge band saw is used on amputated legs and arms to cut sections of tumours when the leg or arm arrives in the pathology department. This is scientifically important for determining the degree of spread of certain tumours. It is a deadly piece of equipment and extreme care needs to be taken when using it. One common rookie mistake is sawing through an arm or a leg before X-raying it . . .

We once had to work on a leg that had been amputated due to a tumour. The leg had a metal rod lodged within the medullary bone cavity. (The medullary cavity is the central cavity of the bone shaft, where orthopaedic surgeons place metal rods after a bone fracture.) No one was aware of the metal rod, because it could not be seen without an X-ray. Imagine sawing a leg or an arm and the serrated wheel blade strikes that metal rod. The blade will instantaneously become blunt (it costs vast amounts of money to replace) and the leg could fly across the pathology laboratory, injuring or even killing oneself or one's technical assistants. Luckily, in this case, the X-rays arrived in the nick of time – literally moments before the amputated leg would have been sawed.

The same goes for oscillating head saws and the neurosurgical screws on the skull. Often, neurosurgeons place metal screws on the skull bone; if an oscillating saw hits one of these screws, it could cause major trouble.

A lesson I have learnt the hard way is that the corpse of a homeless person needs special care. One day, when I was newly qualified, I performed an autopsy on a homeless woman who had died fairly recently. There were so many ticks, fleas and lice on her that it looked like her skin was covered with sand. During the autopsy, several of these jumped onto me.

Even though I was wearing full personal protective equipment and a bouffant, I could not help but feel itchy.

You might wonder why we don't spray such corpses with insecticide. Forensic toxicology machines are so sensitive that they will pick up trace amounts of insecticides in the blood even after death.

And so I learnt to refrigerate homeless people for two to three days before doing an autopsy on them. The cold air kills the ticks, fleas and lice, and makes for an itch-free autopsy.

Exhumation is another rather grisly job that may be expected of forensic pathologists. Over the years, I have been involved in a number of exhumations, which are not the easiest jobs in the world, I must admit.

Once, the body of a woman was found burning on the side of the road in a small rural town outside a large South African city. The local doctor performed a rudimentary autopsy and certified the cause of the death as 'death by fire'. He found an earring on the burned remains. The deceased was never formally identified, and was consequently given a pauper's burial.

Shortly afterwards, there were news reports that the deceased had been a whistle-blower who had been involved with high-level fraud. The story went that she had been murdered and then set alight on the side of the road. This case became very high profile and many questions were being asked. Eventually, it was decided to perform an exhumation.

When we arrived at the paupers' graveyard, it was difficult to determine which grave was hers. The graveyard manager knew that she had been buried in a certain row, but could not identify her grave site. This meant that we had to open all the graves in that specific row.

We began at 6 a.m. and finally finished at 4 p.m. The paupers' graveyard was in an area with a rising and lowering water table, and many of the graves had water damage, making our job even more difficult.

Literally the last grave site in the row turned out to be that of the deceased woman. The next morning, the redo autopsy was performed. The other earring was located and the cause of death was determined – she had been strangled. We also established that she had been set alight after she had been murdered: no soot remains were found in her trachea, indicating that it had not been a death by fire.

The woman was also formally identified by means of her dental work. Fortunately, her family had her dental records, which were then compared with her remains.

The logistics behind this case were quite unbelievable. We had to hire digging equipment and twelve assistants to help unearth the remains. All the other pauper's graves were carefully and respectfully reburied.

The lesson learnt in this specific scenario was that you get one bite at the cherry. Performing an exhumation is an extremely labour-intensive, inconvenient and costly exercise, which must be avoided if at all possible.

In another instance, I was asked to drive to the site of an exhumation in the middle of nowhere, near a river. The forensic team had been digging for hours after a murderer had confessed and pointed out to the police where he had buried his victim. I remember this case very well because it was rocky terrain and my poor car got damaged when I drove over a concealed tree stump.

In a relatively shallow grave the decomposed remains of a man were found, as well as his amputated index finger, which had been buried with him. Apparently the murderer had killed the man and put him in the boot of his car, and had amputated his right index finger to use it to exit the fingerprint-access complex where the man stayed.

In a third case, I was presented with the skeletonised remains of a hand. The human hand has twenty-seven bones, but this one had twenty-three. Apparently it had been found lying beside a dam. Five years earlier, a drug addict walking past the dam found the hand with a ring on the ring finger. He had stolen the ring, presumably for drug money. Five years later he told his girlfriend about the ring. She went to report it to the police. The police then went to the dam and found the remains of the hand.

Now, when examining skeletal remains you have to ask yourself certain questions. For example, are they human bones? From which part of the body are the bones? Are they from a male or a female? How old are they?

My first question was whether or not they were human bones: you would be surprised by what members of the public bring to the mortuary for examination. In the majority of instances where the public or members of the police arrive at the mortuary with a bone, it is from an animal; sometimes, it's even wood or plastic!

What made this case so fascinating was that the skeletonised remains of a baboon were found approximately fifty metres from the skeletonised hand bones, deep in the bushes. However, this baboon had both its hands. And, of course, the fact that a ring was found on the skeletonised hand bones made us suspect that they were human.

DNA examination plays a vital part in such cases. This case was linked to a murder case from ten years before, in which the hand of the victim had been cut off. A decade later, the loop could finally be closed.

In another instance, an innocent night out at a restaurant led to a local and international investigation into a skeleton. That night, the restaurant owner told me that her sister was a teacher who had moved overseas. Apparently she had left an anatomical teaching skeleton behind, which had been used in the school where she had taught. The owner of the restaurant wanted to know what she should do with the skeleton, which at that point was lying in a box in her parents' house.

I discussed this matter with colleagues and was told to phone the police immediately, since no member of the public is allowed to have human tissue in their possession. After the police investigation was launched, they descended upon the parents' house. The house was thoroughly examined and their garden was excavated. The woman's parents were interrogated for some eighteen hours. Her sister was also detained overseas and questioned by local authorities.

What is more, a full skeletal autopsy and DNA testing were performed. It was established that the skeleton had indeed been donated for scientific purposes. This matter cost a lot of time and money, but it was a process we had to go through.

Needless to say, I was never formally invited back to the restaurant again.

4

Time since death

A few years ago a male patient, who had been admitted for a chest condition, disappeared from one of the big academic hospitals. He had not signed a form to indicate his refusing hospital treatment and none of the other patients in the ward nor any of the security guards had any idea what had happened to him.

There were many media reports and much hype about this matter. Three weeks later, the man was found dead in the ceiling of the hospital with a cigarette butt next to him. Clearly, he had sneaked up into the ceiling to have a secret smoke.

What made this particular case so memorable to me was that the body, on which I performed the autopsy, looked like a cotton wool puff ball – it was literally covered in white mould. One would hardly imagine that a human body was at the centre of it. When I finally managed to remove all the mould, I found a scrawny 45 kg man. I performed a thorough autopsy and the cause of death was tuberculosis of the lungs.

Besides the poor pay, decomposition and cases like this are probably the chief factor that stops potential medical practitioners from entering the field of forensic pathology. Practising forensic pathology on the African continent means constant exposure to a relatively large number of decomposed bodies. The African sun is harsh, and bodies are not always found immediately.

One dead body may contain about 70 kg of larvae and maggots. The heat radiating off the maggot mass may be so intense that you can feel it through your apron. One particularly decomposed case had so-called jumping larvae feeding off it. One such larval species jumped off the corpse and into my boot, where it clung to my sock. Later that day, when I undressed, the larval species inch-wormed itself very slowly off my sock!

It always breaks my heart when I get a call about someone who has been found dead in their house, apartment or flat and we arrive to find them severely decomposed. It astounds me just how many people have no support system or infrastructure. It is always the landlord or landlady who finds the body, or the cleaning personnel – rarely a family member.

Decomposition may seem like a nasty mess to an untrained person. Your senses are usually overwhelmed by the putrefaction and decay of a decomposed body. For starters, there's the smell, which some describe as ammonia-like and others as smelling like gorgonzola cheese.

In a decomposed body the abdomen and the external genitalia swell, as well as the tongue, which sticks out between the teeth. The eyes protrude. In places skin slippage is present, and there may also be marbling of the skin, caused by postmortem dilation of the blood vessels. There are multiple blisters on the skin, which are filled with clear fluid. Purging is present from the nostrils and mouth, which often fools rookie police officers into thinking that the deceased had drunk dark-coloured liquid poison – or they mistake it for internal bleeding.

Initial decay occurs during the first thirty-six to seventy-two hours after death. We call this period autolysis. Early or so-called green putrefaction occurs up to one week after death, when the skin generally takes on a green hue. Black putrefaction occurs about one month after death, and butyric fermentation after about two months. At this point, the body has a mature cheese-like smell.

You get dry decay and skeletonisation, as well as mummification, if the corpse is found in a hot, dry environment. Under certain conditions, you may get adipocere formation, where a soap-like layer forms on the outside of the corpse, specifically if the corpse is found in a warm, damp environment. For forensic pathologists, adipocere formation is a good thing, since it almost perfectly preserves all the organs of the deceased. You may even find the last meal in the stomach of the deceased, despite the body having been dead for years.

When one cuts into the tensely distended abdomen of a decomposed body, lots of methane and other gases escape from the peritoneal cavity. This smell is also very characteristic. The gas build-up in the abdomen is so intense that it may cause pressure on the stomach and cause the victim to vomit (which we call purging). It may also be so intense that it places pressure on a pregnant uterus and a (dead) baby may be delivered after the mother's death.

Regarding entomology, there is faunal succession of insects on the body – you will typically find eggs, larvae and puparia. This is the domain of the experienced, full-time specialist in forensic entomology. There are the necrophagous species – invertebrates that feed on the corpse itself. Then there are predators and parasites of the necrophagous species – these species do not feed directly on the corpse. There are also omnivorous species – species that feed on everything. And finally, to complicate matters even further, there are adventive or opportunistic species. These insects simply use the corpse as shelter or a nest.

Maggots help forensic pathologists a lot during an autopsy. So-called maggot masses give us a clue as to the position of original wounds. For example, flies tend to lay their eggs within knife wounds, which can help us to identify them.

As mentioned earlier, there can be up to 70 kg of worms and larvae present in a body. Their activity even produces a crackling or popping sound. If someone dies from cocaine overdose, the body is only found months later and there are multiple larvae present within the body, the larvae tend to be large and hyperactive (from the cocaine). We call these hyperactive larvae super larvae.

One common myth is that hair and nails grow after death. What actually happens is that the body dries up, and it appears as if the hair and nails have grown, whereas in fact the skin has shrunk.

We like to think of ourselves as acute pathologists because we want to do an autopsy as soon after death as possible, since the evidence we find on the body will be better, but this isn't always possible. Fortunately, science is a wonderful thing; we are trained to determine time of death and cause of death even in the most decayed bodies.

If you patiently examine a decomposed body with the same diligence and respect that you would give a fresh body, the results may surprise you. Even the most decomposed brain (which looks like grey toothpaste after long decomposition) may deliver surprising results. When you place a dollop of the grey, sludgy, decomposing brain tissue under the microscope, you may be surprised to still see individual neurons. This is why it takes a special kind of person to practise forensics.

There are many factors that may accelerate or retard the normal rate of decomposition of a human body after death, but thankfully not all autopsied bodies are badly decomposed. The majority are, in fact, relatively fresh.

When forensic pathologists are summoned to the scene of a death, they are required to determine time since death. Diagnosing time since death may have far-reaching medicolegal consequences, which is why it plays such a major role in forensic medicine and forensic pathology. For example, if one finds a body in a field with a gunshot wound and the body appears freshly dead, it would raise many questions if the suspects claim that they shot the victim one week before.

As with all things in life, establishing time since death (thanatology) is quite a complex field, and not an exact science. Many factors can disrupt our findings. For example, if someone is murdered and placed in a freezer, and then dumped at a secondary scene years later, the refrigeration will confound our diagnosis of time since death. The advent of refrigeration theoretically nullifies the entire field of time since death.

Stories abound of primitive people found relatively well-preserved in permafrost. There are even stories of perfectly preserved smallpox and influenza virus genomes found in those who were buried in permafrost.

Establishing time since death may be extremely difficult, but if you know what happens to a normal body after death the battle is half won. Allow me to take you through the process.

Immediately upon death, there is unconsciousness, loss of all reflexes and no reaction to painful stimuli. All muscle tone is lost, though muscles are physically capable of contraction for many hours after death – by means of external electrical stimulation, for example.

The eye is a good place to look for signs of death. These include loss of corneal and light reflexes leading to insensitive corneas and fixed, unreactive pupils. Though the iris responds to chemical stimulation (by atropine, for example) for hours after death, the light reflex is lost as soon as brainstem nuclei suffer ischaemic failure (decreased oxygenation).

The pupils usually assume a mid-dilated position, which is the relaxed neutral position of the pupillary muscle, although they could change their position. You could find a marked difference in the degree of dilation of each pupil, but this has no significance as a diagnostic sign either of a brain lesion or of a drug intoxication. In conditions such as morphine poisoning, where the pupils may be contracted during life, death may allow this to persist or the pupils may dilate to the 'cadaveric position'.

The eye globe tension decreases rapidly, as it depends on arterial pressure for its maintenance. The eyeball feels progressively softer within minutes and the cornea soon loses its glistening reflectivity. The eyelids usually close, unless the flaccid muscles fail to produce the full occlusion that occurs in voluntary closure. Where the sclerae remain exposed, two yellow horizontal lines of desiccated discoloration appear on each side of the cornea within a few hours, becoming brown and then sometimes black. This condition is known as *tache noire*.

When viewed with an ophthalmoscope, the retina provides the earliest positive signs of death when the 'cattle-trucking' of blood in the retinal vessels takes place. At this point, loss of blood pressure causes the blood to break up into segments. This happens all over the body, but it can be seen directly only in the retina.

The ear is also an excellent place to diagnose death. When cold water is squirted into the ears of a dead person, the eyes will show no signs of nystagmus (the eyes normally move from side to side). Make sure that there is no wax in the ears!

Once, I was called to an apartment to ascertain time since death of a young man. His mother was a nursing sister, which meant that she had some background knowledge on the topic. The young man was an invalid and his mother had cared for him for about fourteen years. We discovered a body that had been dead for several months, and was mummified. The mother refused to believe that her son was dead. When I syringed water into the deceased's ear canals to prove that there was no oculocaloric reflex, the mother cried out: 'Look, his eyes moved!' She had even heated the room with a heater to obfuscate the body temperature measurements of the son. The next moment she said, 'There is wax in his ears.'

The mother was in such a state of denial that she even fed her mummified son soup in front of me and my team. This was a most challenging situation. Eventually we had to perform an electrocardiogram or ECG (heart testing) and an electroencephalogram or EEG (brain testing) to prove to her that her son was really dead. The mother remained in denial; eventually, we had to consult social workers, religious leaders, psychologists and psychiatrists.

Diagnosing death can be extremely difficult. I have been fooled; even my senior colleagues have been fooled.

The primary marker of death is when someone's heart stops beating and respiratory movements cease. Cardiac arrest can be determined by prolonged auscultation of the chest to exclude heart sounds, although a feeble heartbeat may be muffled by a thick chest wall or chronic obstructive airway disease (for example, in people who have smoked cigarettes for years). The ECG still remains unchallenged in confirming cardiac arrest.

Respiration is more difficult to confirm, especially in deep coma such as that which accompanies barbiturate poisoning. It may become necessary to place a stethoscope over the trachea or lung fields and listen for a prolonged period. Archaic methods like placing saucers of water on someone's chest or feathers before their nostrils are of historical interest alone.

To determine time since death scientifically, you can use any of the following techniques: supravital reactions, body temperature, rigidity (rigor mortis), lividity (livor mortis), potassium concentrations in the vitreous of the eye, putrefaction changes and entomology. Let me explain a few.

The intermediate period after death is known as the supravital period. External stimuli to the corpse may be life-mimicking for as many as twelve to fifteen hours after death. Supravital reactions include tendon reactions, such as Zsako's phenomenon: if you strike the lower third of the thigh, there is a curious upward movement of the patella (kneecap bone). This may happen two to three hours after death. If you strike the biceps muscle with a reflex hammer, a localised muscular contraction (bulge) at the point of stimulation may be observed. This phenomenon persists for several hours after Zsako's phenomenon.

After death the body cools until it reaches the temperature of its surroundings, also called algor mortis. This takes about eight to twelve hours at the skin surface, with the core of the body taking approximately three times longer. As a rule of thumb, the human body tends to lose 1 °C per hour during the first twenty-four hours. However, this is not a linear function: there is a lag period of half an hour to three hours during the initial phase. In the intermediate phase, however, the temperature drops linearly, and during the terminal phase the body temperature drop slows as the core temperature approaches that of the environment.

The best estimator of time since death during the first twenty-four hours is gained by measuring the core temperature of the body. Obviously, all measurements assume that the deceased died at normal body temperature. If the person had a high fever before death, then the determination of time since death, based on temperature measurement, will be wrong.

We also have cooling equations that help us determine time since death. These cooling equations are even available as nomograms and apps for mobile phones. We just need to be aware of hypothermia as a death mimic.

Using body temperature to determine time since death requires a deep understanding of thermodynamics. There are so many variables that may affect the final answer. But body temperature does give a rough estimation of time since death.

Rigidity or rigor mortis is the normal stiffening of the body after death, which typically begins three to four hours after death. It becomes fully established within about eight to twelve hours. It is due to complex physicochemical changes that occur in muscle proteins after death, including conversion of muscle glycogen to lactic acid. Rigor mortis remains unchanged for about thirty-six hours, and usually disappears within two to three days. Thereafter, secondary flaccidity ensues.

Cadaveric spasm is an interesting rigor mortis-type phenomenon. Often, one finds a corpse clutching something in the hand, making many people believe that the person held on to that object when they died and that rigor mortis set in immediately. This is not so, given that rigor mortis typically takes about three or more hours to set in. Cadaveric spasm appears to be a rare form of instantaneous rigor that develops at the time of death with no period of post-mortem flaccidity. It seems confined to deaths that took place in the midst of intense physical and/or emotional activity. This phenomenon usually affects one group of muscles, such as the flexors of the arm, rather than the whole body. Most cases of cadaveric spasm occur in similar circumstances; it is said to be common among soldiers slain in combat. There remains much controversy surrounding this condition.

Lividity is also known as hypostasis or plurifocal staining of the skin. It is caused by the gravitational settling of blood in the body of a dead person. Lividity depends on the posture of the corpse at death. It does not appear on areas exposed to pressure, so if the person is found dead on his back, you will not see death staining on the shoulder blades and buttocks. It is perceptible within about three to four hours, and is at its peak approximately eight to twelve hours after death.

During this period, lividity is still mobile – in other words, it may be moved by applying pressure to the deceased's skin with one's finger (except in cases where someone died from major bleeding). After about twelve to fifteen hours, the lividity becomes fixed. The phenomenon of lividity generally lends itself to subjective interpretation.

None of the aforementioned methods of determining time since death are foolproof. Temperature measurement is probably the most scientific method currently in use. Measurement of the potassium concentration within the fluid compartment of the eyes is a very useful method. External examination of lividity and rigidity are also regularly used, as is electrical excitability of facial muscles and chemical excitability of the iris.

When all is said and done, we as forensic pathologists can at most give a broad estimate of time of death. We can tell the courts that a victim died between three and six hours before the body was discovered. If you ever hear someone say, 'My Lord, death occurred yesterday at exactly 2:33 p.m.,' you should be sceptical.[10]

5

African wildlife deaths

Africa is a place of unimaginable beauty, but it is also a place of unimaginable hardship and danger. There are dangerous wild animals such as lions, crocodiles and hippopotami to contend with, not to mention the reptiles: the Cape cobra and black mamba are the snakes responsible for the most deaths in Southern Africa. And then there are mosquitoes and malaria.

The weather on the continent also keeps things wild and untamed. Thunderstorms are a regular occurrence, so forensic pathologists see a host of lightning-related deaths.

If you drive around rural Africa, the first thing that could strike you – literally and figuratively – is the large number of free-ranging cattle, goats and donkeys on the roads. These wandering, foraging beasts regularly cause accidental deaths on the continent. Wild animals are also notorious for being hit by cars at night in Africa. I know of several cases of cars striking hippopotami and kudu.

In the coastal regions we see shark attacks, deaths related to scuba diving and even deaths caused by other marine creatures. My colleague once had to do an autopsy on someone who had died while scuba diving. The body arrived at the mortuary still in the wetsuit. What did he find inside it?

A dead scorpionfish, one of the most poisonous species in the ocean.

Due to the vast, open spaces on the continent, it is not uncommon for people to be murdered or bodies to be dumped in wilderness areas. Refugees who try to enter the country through our cross-border game reserves have been attacked by wild animals.

You never know what kind of cases will be on the cutting list on any particular day if you are a forensic pathologist in Africa. Medicolegal autopsies are often performed by doctors in the periphery with no formal or official training in forensic pathology. They may be retired district surgeons who have trained themselves on how to perform autopsies, or general practitioners with an interest in forensic pathology.

In the more rural parts of South Africa and the rest of the continent there may be no formal forensic infrastructure at all, and the local GP may have to perform an autopsy out of pure necessity. Lack of resources makes this a relatively widespread and inevitable practice in many developing countries. This is detrimental to the high standard of expertise that is vital for the support of law enforcement and administration of justice.

Practising forensics in Africa can be extremely challenging at the best of times. The real problems are highlighted when an overseas tourist dies an unnatural death somewhere on the continent and the family demands the same level of excellence that are reached in many developed countries.

Forensic pathologists who work on the continent are often at personal risk. There have been cases of forensic pathologists who have simply disappeared after finding something contrary to some or other government agency. The International Day of the Disappeared on 30 August is intended to draw attention to the fate of such individuals and those imprisoned under poor conditions in places that are often unknown to their relatives and/or legal representatives.[11]

Working as a forensic pathologist in a developing country brings its own set of challenges. For instance, one Monday morning when I arrived at work, the mortuary had no water. As I have explained, water is absolutely essential for performing medicolegal autopsies.

The body of a 70 kg man contains approximately five litres of blood. One needs constantly flowing water to rinse away blood and seek out the pathology.

On this particular day, we had to be flexible and do what we could with what we had available. We emptied large municipal bins and got the fire department to fill the bins with water. We used sixteen fifty-litre municipal bins to perform autopsies on twelve bodies.

Blood also stains, and it is incredibly difficult to remove these stains. You really have to scrub floors to remove blood. Dried blood also adheres to the skin and requires extreme scrubbing to remove. Dried blood in a skin fold on the hand of a deceased may look like an incised defence wound. We therefore need to thoroughly scrub the bodies down to find injuries and get decent photographs of the pathological conditions.

While we're on the topic of blood, the fact that blood is so difficult to get rid of is a helpful tool for forensic investigators. Luminol is a white to pale-yellow crystalline solid that is soluble in most polar organic solvents, but insoluble in water. Forensic investigators use luminol to detect trace amounts of blood at crime scenes, as it reacts with the iron in haemoglobin.

Because the blood is only acting as a catalyst, small traces that are invisible to the eye are sufficient to trigger the reaction, so luminol can be used to detect blood spatter and pools even after cleaning. When luminol is sprayed evenly across an area, trace amounts of an activating oxidant make the luminol emit a blue glow that is visible in a darkened room.

It is also not uncommon to arrive at the mortuary to find that there is no electricity due to load shedding or cable theft. At times, the oscillating head saws are broken, which means having to use manual hacksaws to open the skulls, or we could be out of insect spray, leaving the mortuary buzzing with thousands of flies. There may be no personal protective equipment, or there may be labour relations issues.

You never know what a day at the mortuary may bring. For this reason, you always have to be flexible and you should have a positive attitude. And, most importantly, when the moment calls for it, you must be resilient and able to make a plan.

Another scourge of African mortuaries is flies, especially in the summer months. Flies are part and parcel of being a forensic pathologist in Africa. If you are squeamish about flies, this job is probably not for you. A memory comes to mind of a fly, taking off sluggishly from a decomposing corpse and striking my neck before falling into my disposable gown and surgical scrubs, and under my shirt. The next moment it was flying around inside my shirt, but my hands were gloved and covered with blood. Calmly, I had to de-glove and begin the ritual of first removing my protective gear before I could try to free the fly from inside my neatly tucked clothing.

Over the years, we have tried every single tactic to rid mortuaries of flies. We have installed fly screens, fancy ultraviolet fly-attracting and electrical fly-shocking devices, and have placed foul-smelling concoctions in fly traps in and around the mortuary. We have tried every brand and make of insecticide, except for DDT, to try to halt what is known as blowfly invasion. One colleague took a two-litre cola bottle and drilled 6 mm holes into the sides before placing a piece of rotting fish inside, to which the flies took immediately. Despite all these crafty methods, the flies still manage to find their way into the mortuary.

Flies are not all bad, though. Sometimes they are our friends. Once, a fly helped me make the diagnosis at autopsy when it landed on an organ and died on the spot. It turned out the deceased had committed suicide by ingesting an insecticide.

When we're not dealing with flies, we have to watch out for rats. Every now and again, a rat will sneak into the mortuary or arrive on a death scene and cause, for lack of a better word, trouble. Rats like to eat the soft body parts of human bodies, such as the ear lobes, the nose, the tips of the fingers, the toes and the external genitalia. They also have a taste for the wires of C-arms and X-ray machines, and tend to destroy these machines.

In Africa, rats regularly predate on dead humans. I have seen the effects of the black rat (*Rattus rattus*, otherwise known as the ship rat, roof rat or house rat) and the brown rat (*Rattus norvegicus*), both omnivores. Rats are also vectors for disease transmission because they can carry bacteria and viruses in their systems.

Over the years, I have asked numerous pest control experts how to control the scourge that is the rat. Despite all the correct and appropriate occupational health and safety procedures, rats *will* find a way in, even at a state-of-the-art mortuary. They are very crafty and they often avoid the poisons and traps you set out for them. I have seen rats that regurgitate poisons and rats that have become resistant to certain poisons.

The rat is prey to cats and owls, which is why you want to avoid using rat poisons. You do not inadvertently want to poison owls and cats who feed on the dead rats. So, how do you control rats? Certain experts have advocated a 'one-kill' poison that kills the rat at the point of contact with the poison. A shoebox with a rat-sized hole in it containing a one-kill poison is probably advocated. I am a forensic pathologist and not a pest control expert. However, in a resource-limited and resource-depleted environment, one may at times be forced to act beyond one's responsibilities and abilities.

Years of experience suggest that rats love certain brands of sherry and also peanut butter. The pest control expert will try to get the rat addicted to the sherry by placing a single bottle cap in the roof. A few weeks later, the rat expert will lace the sherry with a one-kill rat poison. This method has also been tried, with some success, with peanut butter.

Be that as it may, rats continue to be a scourge in the African forensic setting and they are becoming cleverer, craftier and bigger. When you think you are rat free, think again!

Forensic pathologists who work on the African continent are also involved with wildlife-related human deaths, some of which may be quite dramatic. I have been directly and indirectly involved in doing autopsies on three lion-related deaths, three ostrich-related deaths, one blesbok-related death, three black mamba deaths and two deaths caused by elephants. I have also done autopsies on multiple honey-bee-related cases; fatal dog-bite cases; and horse- and cattle-related cases.

In *Death in the Long Grass*, Peter Hathaway Capstick tells of lions who kill humans for mere folly. He tells how, one day, when one of Kenya's top game rangers was driving in a game reserve with his wife and young son, a lion sprang into the open vehicle. It grabbed the boy by the skull and dragged him out of the Land Rover, severely mauling him until, somehow, the father was able to reclaim his son. The boy survived, although some brain damage was suspected.[12]

Capstick also discussed an incident that took place in 1972 in the Wankie Game Reserve (now the Hwange National Park) in Zimbabwe, where lions gave two families a night of indescribable horror. Over a two-day period, three lions had become increasingly bold, even to the point of entering the camp and eating chickens belonging to the staff. One night, a big lioness leaped through the window of a hut, grabbed one of the women by the small of her back and shook her. It then went on to attack one of the men.

I struggled to believe both of these stories until I had a similar case myself. It involved a young boy who was on a safari camp in a local park. At some point he went into the communal kitchen where he was attacked by a lioness that had apparently leaped through the open window. It grabbed the boy by the head, shook him and fractured his neck. He survived – but succumbed, several days later, in hospital.

The other lion-related deaths involved tourists who were at a farm where tourists can pet lion cubs. Two tourists were accidentally scratched by the lion cubs. They contracted *Bartonella henselae* infection and died from cat scratch disease, a deadly bacterial infection.

A clinical colleague of mine, Ralf, once dealt with a case in which a couple were attacked by a male ostrich in Barberton. The ostrich, which had bright red shins and was full of testosterone, attacked both of them when they crossed a field. Its claw penetrated the woman's stomach and disembowelled her. After a kick to her stomach, she had partial evisceration of the abdomen and a broken femur. The man was kicked in the face, with resultant facial fractures. Both victims survived.

In another ostrich-related case, a forensic pathologist colleague performed the autopsy on a farm worker who was trampled by a male ostrich. The farm worker died from multiple directed blunt force trauma injuries to the body.

As mentioned earlier, a blesbok once killed a worker at a game auction when its horn went through his right nostril and brain, then fractured through his skull. He was trying to transport the blesbok when the accident happened.

The first dead body I ever saw was when I travelled to Hwange National Park as a teenager with my family and another family. The incident occurred on a Sunday on a sunset drive. Our game ranger, who was thirty-six years old at the time, was attacked and killed by an adult elephant. The mother elephant became aggressive and charged him. He tried to chase the elephant away but was gored to death. I was too young to recall all the circumstances leading up to the death, but I do recall having seen the dead body. One of the elephant's tusks had penetrated the man's abdomen, and the elephant had also knelt on him.

In another case involving an elephant, a guide sustained multiple directed blunt force trauma injuries when he was attacked. He survived for a few weeks, but died in hospital. I was consulted forensically about this case.

There is nothing more chilling than coming face to face with a black mamba when walking through the African bushveld. These venomous snakes, which are found in Southern Africa, can raise themselves off the ground to almost adult height. Their heads are shaped like a coffin, their eyes look like lifeless, black beads, and they have neurotoxic (and cardiotoxic) venom. Despite their name, they are usually dark brown, olive-brown or gunmetal in colour.

I have investigated three black mamba deaths so far in my career. The first involved a twelve-year-old girl from Phalaborwa who was bitten on the thigh when she was walking on a dirt road and came across a black mamba. At the time, I was still working as a doctor at the Maphuthi Malatji Hospital. She died in my arms at the hospital.

The second involved a tourist who visited a snake park in one of our northern provinces. The snake park employees were showing him a baby black mamba when it accidentally fell out of its glass jar and onto his hand. He must have been bitten by the snake, since he died a few minutes later.

The third case concerned a man who was doing snake venom extraction at a venom extraction facility in Gauteng. Post extraction, a single fang from a black mamba hooked on

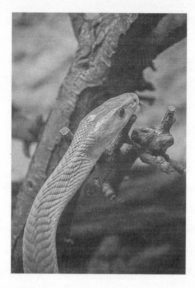

A black mamba.
Photo: T Birkenbach

his index finger and he, too, died. I have also heard of a case in which a black mamba was flushed and killed by a pack of inexperienced dogs. Four or more of the dogs were bitten in rapid succession, and died before the snake could be torn to pieces.

The maximum venom yield of a large black mamba is often given as 400 mg, but it is probably closer to 280 mg. Approximately 15–20 mg of venom is required for a bite to be fatal to a human. The black mamba is born with approximately two to three drops of venom per fang (adults have twelve to twenty drops per fang) but only two drops of venom are required to kill an adult human, making even the young black mamba a very dangerous snake.

Of all Africa's venomous snakes, the black mamba is the largest and most feared. It is of somewhat uncertain temper and often displays great truculence and readiness to attack if suddenly disturbed or otherwise molested. This readiness to attack is particularly evident during the mating season – spring or early summer – when it is more irritable and aggressive than usual. Although this snake has a reputation for being the most dangerous in Africa, it is actually shy and elusive, and generally tries to avoid humans.

Southern Africa loses about six to ten people a year due to bee stings. The western or European honey bee is the most common of the seven species of honey bee worldwide.

While for most people a bee sting is painful or otherwise relatively harmless, in people with insect sting allergy a sting may trigger a dangerous anaphylactic reaction. This is a serious allergic reaction that is rapid in onset and may cause death. In addition, honey bee stings may cause the bees to release pheromones that prompt other nearby bees to attack.

Of the six honey-bee-related deaths I have come across so far, one case involved a member of the clergy who sustained a single bee sting to his forehead. He died due to coronary artery plaque rupture, which led to a heart attack.

Another case involved a single bee sting in a young person that led to a massive anaphylactic reaction. Anaphylaxis typically causes more than one of the following: an itchy rash, throat or tongue swelling, shortness of breath, vomiting, light-headedness, and low blood pressure. These symptoms typically come on over minutes.

Then there was the middle-aged woman who went to walk her dog in the late afternoon in her suburb. No one knows what provoked it, but a swarm of bees attacked the woman and her dog. When the body of the woman arrived at the mortuary, she was literally covered in thousands of bee stings. The bees had also killed her dog. They had stung the woman through her jeans, in her eyes and even inside her nostrils. I had never seen anything like it.

South Africa also has dangerous marine animals – think sharks and stingrays. Since I live inland, I have not had the opportunity to perform any autopsies on shark-related deaths, although many of my forensic colleagues who live on the coast have.

Africa's inland rivers and lakes are filled with many different kinds of fish, catfish and crabs, most of which tend to feed on dead humans. There are almost always post-mortem predation injuries on bodies found in or near fresh water.

A crocodile death that is forever etched in my memory was recounted to me by my good friend Bryan when I was practising medicine in Phalaborwa. One day, when I visited him at his girlfriend's house, I noticed a photograph of another man, about Bryan's age, on the mantelpiece. When I asked them who the fellow was, Bryan's girlfriend's eyes welled up with tears. They told me the story. A group of friends, including the nineteen-year-old in the photograph, had gone camping near the Oliphants River near Phalaborwa. At some point, they had all gone swimming in the river. The man had screamed, '*Iets byt my!* (Something is biting me!)' and then disappeared under the water.

He had been taken by a crocodile. The chilling thing is that they never found his body. Even years later, no skeletal remains have been found.

Another very sad story is of one of my medical colleagues who owned a crocodile farm. One day, as he was feeding his crocodiles, he slipped and fell into the water. The crocodiles attacked and killed him.

Stories about attacks by dangerous African wildlife and deaths caused by these animals have always gripped people's imagination. They are horrified at the thought of the pain of a lion attack or the helplessness of being pulled underwater by a crocodile. However, I have good news – these deaths are extremely rare. In the greater scheme of things, and when you look at the statistics, the chances of dying in your car on your way to buy a lottery ticket are greater than your chances of being killed by a wild animal – or of actually winning the lottery! The chances of dying as a result of diabetes mellitus, smoking or in a pedestrian vehicle accident are far greater than dying by a man-eating wild animal.

No book that deals with animal and insect-related deaths on the African continent will be complete without mentioning malaria. Malignant cerebral malaria is caused by the parasite *Plasmodium falciparum*. It continues to afflict about 200 million patients each year, killing more than 600 000.

Malaria is probably one of the biggest talking points for overseas visitors on safari in Africa. And when it comes to malaria, everyone seems to be an expert. The history of the discovery of malaria and its treatment is a long one, with many great names. Many visitors arrive here with a homeopathic antimalarial agent or herbal tincture that has not passed the rigorous controls of modern-day science. Their citronella oil sprays only serve to excite the local hyper-testosteronised elephant populations. Sadly, these people often contract malaria – and some even die.

While malaria is often the first thing people think about when travelling to Africa, it is usually the last thing they think about twenty-one days after returning from a visit to the continent. Due to malaria's twenty-one-day incubation period, people totally forget causality in this regard and falsely attribute their flu-like symptoms or their headache to something unrelated. Malaria is a natural death, yet on the table of a forensic pathologist it often presents as an unnatural one. The simple reason is that malaria victims are often found dead with little background history. A sudden, unexplained and unexpected death raises questions; the matter becomes suspicious, requiring police investigation.

At autopsy, there are typically no injuries on the body. Internally, you may find an enlarged spleen and the brain appears to be almost purple in colour from being so congested. But the real diagnosis happens under the microscope. There, you notice *Plasmodium falciparum*-infected red cells marginating within veins in the brain, and sometimes the faint birefringent hemozoin pigment and Dürck's granulomas (small focal inflammatory reactions).

One of the strangest malaria deaths I have encountered involved a well-off woman who was found dead in her five-star hotel room. She was naked, in the bathtub.

Now, when people die in a bathtub it often presents a very difficult forensic situation. If you consider the normal bathroom, there are slippery surfaces on which people could slip and injure their heads. They may have overdosed on medication, or have been electrocuted. Some bathrooms have gas geysers, with which people could gas themselves. And, of course, you could drown in a bath full of water (in an accident, suicide, or homicide, or through natural causes).

However, after a thorough post-mortem examination, we finally established that the woman had died of cerebral malaria. Apparently, she had visited a game reserve in a neighbouring African country twenty-one days before . . .

6

Lightning and environmental deaths

People travel to the northern hemisphere and pay lots of money to see the Northern Lights. However, to my mind there are few things as dramatic or astonishing as an electric Highveld summer thunderstorm. As impressive as it can be, lightning is South Africa's biggest weather killer. Each year, eighty to one hundred South Africans die due to lightning, and about seven times as many people get struck and survive.

I once saw a fence that had been struck by lightning. In quite an ironic twist, the metal wire had completely disappeared and only the Viro lock, with signs of lightning on it, remained.

Compared with other places in the world, lightning deaths are relatively common in Africa. People in some parts of Africa have limited access to public transport, so many walk home after work. Thunderstorms typically strike between 15:30 and 18:30 – when people are on their way home.

Furthermore, when it comes to protecting people from lightning, there are limited safe shelters on the continent. What is a safe shelter, you might ask? A suitable shelter may be any fully enclosed metallic surface area, known as a Faraday cage or a Gaussian surface. There is a need for lightning protection

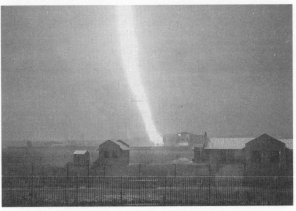

Lightning is powerful and often deadly. *Photo: T Stuart*

systems for small structures in Africa and other developing countries.

I have performed many autopsies on people and animals that have been struck by lightning. Even though I am a forensic pathologist concerned with human deaths, I have dealt with a large number of lightning-related deaths in cows, sheep, wild dogs, elephants, rhinos, giraffes, kestrels, koi fish, whooping cranes, geese and even doves.

I have subsequently become very interested in, and something of an expert on, lightning-related deaths. In fact, I did my doctorate on lightning-related injury mechanisms. The reason I became so fascinated is that the lightning incident occurs with a millisecond. And so much happens within that millisecond that it is almost impossible to observe everything in that short time span.

It requires extreme forensics to try to work out what exactly happened in that momentary flash of brightness – which is why we have to look for clues about what happened on the scene, and on the body.

One of the first lightning-strike cases that captured the collective South African imagination took place in the Free State, near what is today the Golden Gate National Park. There, you'll find two graves side by side. The black marble slabs bear the message, in Afrikaans, that the gravestones are in loving memory of Valerie Wilcocks, born on 23 December 1910, and Johan Bestendig de la Harpe, born 17 December 1911, both of whom were killed by lightning at Mont-aux-Sources on 18 December 1932.

Valerie was a twenty-two-year-old student. Johan was due to celebrate his twenty-first birthday two days later, and was studying for a degree in agriculture at the (now) University of Pretoria. Johan and Valerie were leading Johan's horse when there was a blinding flash of light and a terrific clap of thunder.

Valerie was declared dead immediately. Johan de la Harpe died at midnight.

The two students were laid to rest in the quiet of the hills they so loved. Twelve years later, Carl Wilcocks, Valerie's brother, erected a bronze at the spot where the tragedy happened.[13]

Another terrible lightning incident took place on 11 November 1994 in a rural area near Modimolle (then called Nylstroom). A group of twenty-six ten- and eleven-year-old girls went camping with two adults and seven dogs at the end of a week-long school trip.

Most of the group had been sleeping outside. When light rain started to fall, they decided to move into a ten-by-five-metre tent. No rain had fallen in the area for months, so the floor of the tent was dry. The main supports of the tent were two 3.6 m isolated metal poles at either end, 5 m apart.

Between 2 a.m. and 2:30 a.m., four lightning flashes oc-

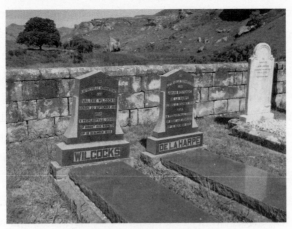

The gravestones of Valerie Wilcocks and Johan Bestendig
de la Harpe (in the van Reenen family cemetery, Golden Gate
National Park). *Photo: S Rossouw*

curred in the vicinity. The adult supervisors were awakened
by a tremendous explosion and the feeling of having had a
shock. The children recalled strong, choking fumes, and the
smell of burned feathers and plastic.

Four children were fatally injured at the time of the strike.
Others had significant injuries. Four of the seven dogs were
also killed. There was no immediate medical care available
to the victims. The closest farmhouse was more than a kilometre away, and the closest medical facility was about eighty
kilometres away. They didn't have a telephone or other means
to call for help.

The incident was investigated by local electrical engineers
AE Carte and Ralph Anderson, and an ER physician from
the USA, Mary Ann Cooper. I met Ralph Anderson seventeen
years later at his retirement home. He was ninety-four at the
time. Over a whisky, he told me about the lightning incident.

He even showed me the tent; lightning had struck one of the poles.

He then pulled out a piece of paper with the names of all the surviving girls written on it. Ralph made me promise that I would do a follow-up study on the incident. He cared greatly; he wanted me to find out how the girls were doing, and whether they had suffered any consequences.

A few months later, I was giving a lecture on lightning in Grahamstown at a science festival. A young girl approached me after the lecture. She identified herself as B and said that she was one of the survivors of the lightning accident near Modimolle. She was in contact on Facebook with all the other girls who had survived.

In 2012, I attended the International Conference on Lightning Protection (ICLP) in Vienna, where I met Mary Ann Cooper. She had travelled to the conference from the USA. I told her that I had met Ralph Anderson and B, and that I had given Ralph my word that I would do a follow-up study of the survivors. There and then, Mary Ann and I agreed to do such a study.

Cooper enrolled two psychologists from the University of Illinois at Chicago. We also had to pass the study by two ethics and integrity committees. We had to respond to very serious considerations at the ethics committees – for example, what if recounting this event would emotionally traumatise these girls a second time and if so, how would we respond?

I also visited the school they had attended and met with the headmistress and the previous headmistress to obtain their respective consent. The daughter of the previous headmistress had died in the incident. Every year, they hold a memorial service at the school for the girls who died.

We designed a research questionnaire and B offered to serve

as a liaison with the surviving group members to assess initial interest from their side. There were twenty-two survivors, many of whom had emigrated and who now lived all over the world. In 2013, we approached them directly via e-mail as the researchers.

What happened next came quite unexpectedly. None of the girls responded to our questionnaire. This led to several e-mails between us and the members of the group.

Finally, one of the girls – let's call her C – told us why this had happened. In an emotional e-mail, she explained that she had informed all the other girls *not* to take part in the study because she couldn't understand why they hadn't had any support in the preceding nineteen years and why now, all of a sudden, we wanted to interview them.

The girls had seen several medical practitioners. These included a wide variety of specialists, from ear, nose and throat (ENT) specialists to occupational therapists and psychologists. The consequence was that they never knew who their 'main' doctor was and felt that no one had really taken responsibility for their long-term health. Many of the girls suffered severe physical and emotional trauma. A close doctor–patient relationship is critical when it comes to lightning-strike patients, which requires lifelong continuity of patient management.

Some of the girls suffered hearing problems, others had eye problems, and a number of them had neurological problems. Most were traumatised by the incident and were terrified of electrical thunderstorms.

I was unsure how to respond to C's e-mail, so I decided to have a cup of tea and think it through. Within the next hour, I read an SABC news report that fourteen construction workers had been sleeping in a tent in the Klarinet informal settlement in Witbank (now Emalahleni) when lightning had struck the tent. Eight of them had died immediately; six others had been injured, and were taken to hospital.

I sent this tragic news article to C and tried to explain that it was incumbent on us to document this incident in the most comprehensive way – and that we were approaching it from a strictly scientific point of view. 'We have to do this from a sense of duty,' I wrote.

By that evening, the entire group of surviving girls had responded to our questionnaire. Twenty-two years after the lightning strike, the follow-up study was published in the *South African Medical Journal*.[14] I had kept my promise to Ralph Anderson, even though he had sadly passed away several months before.

The fact that the girls still keep in contact with one another via social media demonstrates the impact of the 1994 incident on each of their lives. Given the rapid changes in the communication landscape brought about by participative Internet use and social media, it was important to note the importance of these technologies and their impact on health communication.

Our key findings were that there was a paucity of data on the long-term after-effects of lightning strike on survivors. Therefore, the importance of such a study examining both the physical and psychological sequelae of lightning strike could not be understated.

I mentioned that I have also been involved with investigating the deaths of several animals that had died due to lightning. The first case involved a horse that had allegedly been struck by lightning. The skeletonised remains of a mare were discovered on 7 January 2008 on a farm near a large coastal town.

What is important to note in this case is that the horse was insured for a vast sum of money. The mare was allegedly last seen alive on 31 December 2007. It was thought to have been struck by lightning between these two dates.

I had grave reservations about the proposed time of death. In my opinion, the advanced degree of skeletonisation would have taken longer than the seven-day period suggested. Examination of the mare's remains showed no periosteum (a dense layer of connective tissue enveloping the bones) and the bones appeared bleached by sunlight. In my opinion, the remains had probably been lying there for *at least* three weeks. The proposed time of death was therefore highly unlikely.

The horse's owner had suggested lightning as the cause of death, but his timeline was not plausible. The case was therefore deemed to be one of fraud and the vast amount of insurance money was not paid out in the end.

The second case involved a dead sable antelope that was also insured for a vast amount of money. Apparently, the sable antelope had been struck by lightning, after which its owner, a farmer, had had it processed into meat for his workers. The head of the sable was taken to a taxidermist and mounted as a trophy. The farmer then claimed for the insured amount.

The Lightning Network Detection System Data from the South African Weather Service informed us that lightning had indeed been recorded on the farmer's property during the time at which the farmer claimed the animal had been struck. We also examined the antelope's mounted head and found positive signs of lightning on it (one eardrum was indeed ruptured). In the end, the insurance claim was confirmed, based on our findings.

The third case involved two bongos at a South African zoo.

Bongos are an incredibly rare antelope species and each cost in the region of R300 000. After a severe thunderstorm in the vicinity of the zoo in January 2012, the two bongos were found dead in their enclosure. A veterinary pathologist was in charge of the case and I was called due to my interest in lightning deaths.

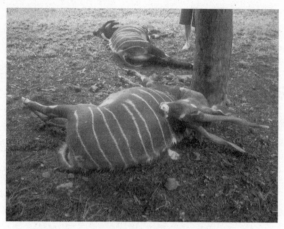

Two bongos were found dead in their enclosure at a South African zoo after a thunderstorm. *Photo: R Blumenthal*

A full autopsy was performed on each bongo. Findings were in keeping with the available history of lightning. Surprisingly, the bongos showed very few external findings, although they did have pinpoint haemorrhages overlying the epicardial surface of the heart and between the fissures of the lungs.

Two electrical engineers, who also studied this incident, came up with a lightning protection plan for critically endangered species at zoos. Their plan won them the best young scientist prize at the International Conference of Lightning Protection, held in Vienna, later that same year.

As one can see from these three stories, the need for

forensic expertise in the veterinary arena appears to be greater now than ever before. In 2013, billionaire businessman Johann Rupert led a group that bought a Cape buffalo bull called Mystery for a record R40 million.[15] This single example shows what is at stake in the veterinary world.

How should one perform a medicolegal autopsy on a R40 million buffalo if it suddenly dropped dead? Imagine performing an autopsy on a R25 million racehorse, or a critically endangered species. Veterinary pathologists have to do this all the time, although some have not had the same rigorous training as human forensic pathologists. With species being insured at such exorbitant amounts, the forensic bar appears to be set higher than ever.

Are human forensic pathology skills transferable to the veterinary disciplines? If so, what is the path forward and what are the ethics involved? Would forensic veterinary pathology ever be considered its own mainstream discipline?

Rhino poaching is a scourge on the continent and stock theft remains a major problem. Poisoning of pets is, and still remains, a heavy burden on pet owners; some people's pets are dearer to them than their own family members. There remains a thriving illegal pet trade. Sudden unexpected deaths of animals will always need a thorough forensic approach. In short, there is definitely a need for forensic veterinary pathology.

Lightning is the cause of another life-threatening phenomenon that is pretty common in South Africa – the veld fire. As forensic pathologists, we often come across deaths that resulted from veld fires. The international term for this phenomenon is 'wildland fires'. These fires can be started by nature herself (lightning) or by man (throwing a cigarette into the dry grass, for example), and can be started accidentally or intentionally (arson).

Wildland fires do not generally contain the toxic compounds produced by plastics and other household materials. They do, however, impair visibility, release carbon monoxide, and carry suspended particulates that may cause severe physical irritation of the lungs. Your senses may be overcome by the sudden darkness, thick and blinding smoke, searing heat and flames as high as two to three metres.

Veld fires can spread incredibly quickly. Rates of 2.3 km/h or 40 m/min have been cited in literature.[16] Fires obviously spread faster up slopes than down slopes. A frontal wind passage may also exacerbate a wildfire.

Veld fires can kill people who get caught in the blaze directly, but can also kill people indirectly. In September 2019, a veld fire took place along a major national highway in Gauteng. Thick, white plumes of smoke hung over the highway, which made drivers slow down. Sadly, a truck, which did not brake in time, ploughed into the back of some of the cars. Multiple people died in this incident.

Veld fires may also open up the grasslands, exposing things that were previously concealed. It is not uncommon for a passerby to discover a burned body in the veld after such a fire. These bodies are then sent to forensic pathology for examination. The cases I have dealt with have varied from homicides, where the bodies have been dumped in the veld, to homeless people, who were sleeping in the veld when the fire overcame them.

7

Every contact leaves a trace

It was Herbert MacDonell who said, 'Physical evidence cannot be intimidated. It does not forget. It sits there and waits to be detected, preserved, evaluated, and explained.' Everything forensic pathologists do, and I really mean *everything* we do, revolves around Locard's principle, otherwise known as the law of interchange. In forensic science, Locard's exchange principle holds that the perpetrator of a crime will bring something into the crime scene and/or leave with something from it, and that both may be used as forensic evidence. In short, every contact leaves a trace.

Edmond Locard (1877–1966), the director of a crime laboratory in Lyon, France, wrote:

> Wherever he steps, whatever he touches, whatever he leaves, even unconsciously, will serve as a silent witness against him. Not only his fingerprints or his footprints, but his hair, the fibres from his clothes, the glass he breaks, the tool mark he leaves, the paint he scratches, the blood or semen he deposits or collects. All of these and more, bear mute witness against him.
>
> This is evidence that does not forget. It is not confused

by the excitement of the moment. It is not absent because human witnesses are. It is factual evidence. Physical evidence cannot be wrong, it cannot perjure itself, it cannot be wholly absent. Only human failure to find it, study and understand it, can diminish its value.[17]

As an example, let us assume that four students arrive late for an examination and claim it was because of a tyre puncture. A medical detective would say, 'That's nice, let us prove this!' A scientifically rigorous medicolegal investigator would go one step further and say, 'That's nice, let us disprove this!'

So how do we go about proving or disproving their claim? First things first. The investigator impounds their car, confiscates their mobile phones and then separates all four students and interrogates them independently.

There are testimonial evidence and physical evidence. As a scientist, you hardly ever believe testimonial evidence unless it is independently provided and corroborates on the smallest of details. Remember, if people are not lying all of the time, they are lying some of the time. If they are not lying all of the time or some of the time, then they are telling you everything *except* the truth. And if they are not telling you everything except the truth, then they are telling you what they believe to be the truth.

As a next step, you would interrogate the students on their testimonial evidence. What time did the tyre puncture take place? Who noticed the tyre puncture first? Which actions were taken? Who took these actions? Did anyone phone for help? Who did they phone? Whose mobile phone did they use?

You can even pretend to have more (or less) knowledge than

you actually have and play the witnesses off against each another. You may even create fake information in an effort to ascertain the truth. This is called information manipulation. Ideally, at the end of the interrogation, all of the students' versions should corroborate one another.

Regarding the physical evidence, the investigators must examine the car for a punctured tyre. Had the tyre been recently plugged or changed? Who did the students phone to report the punctured tyre? Was their number plate registered at the toll gate at the time they were supposed to pass through it? Were their faces recognised by any recognition software? Forensic entomologists may even scrape the bugs off the windscreen to try to determine whether the students travelled at night or during the day, if this is deemed relevant to the investigation.

The testimonial evidence must corroborate the version created in the minds of the investigators from the physical evidence.

When it comes to murder, suicide and accident cases, we apply these same methods. A scene may be broken up into hundreds of different components. We may send the weapon to a ballistics expert for an opinion, and consult soil experts, climatologists and even veterinarians. It all depends on the details of the particular case. In everything, we use science to help solve problems of the law.

Take the following example: A woman died on the operating table because she had accidently received the wrong blood. According to the available history, her death was due to a blood transfusion reaction. This was a case of potential medical negligence, and huge sums of money and professional reputations were at stake.

The only problem was that the empty packets that had contained the wrong blood had mysteriously disappeared, making it very difficult to prove the blood transfusion reaction scientifically. These blood transfusion vaculitres (labelled packets that could have been tested for the type of blood) were critical to the forensic examination. The hospital's rubbish and waste containers were thoroughly searched, yet there was no trace of the packets. There was even talk that they could accidently have been incinerated.

All we had to work with was the deceased woman's body. Somehow, we had to prove that she had received the wrong blood.

After much reading, and keeping Locard's principle in mind, we proceeded to do something that was not really well described in the literature at the time. We went looking for the transfused blood cells from the donated blood packets within the deceased. This basically meant analysing the deceased woman's liver and spleen for sequestrated red blood cell group antigens from the transfused blood. The theory was that if we found foreign blood group antigens sequestrated within the deceased woman's liver or spleen, we could prove that she had received the wrong blood.

We managed to solve this particular case. The science behind it was thrilling.

Two further questions to consider: Does the presence of evidence equal evidence of presence, and does the absence of evidence equal evidence of absence? Just because something is there, does it mean that it really was there, or could it have been planted there? And just because something is not there, does that mean it really was not there, or could it have been purposefully removed?

To practise good forensics, one needs to be something of a sceptic. Let's say a fingerprint is found on a crime scene. Does this mean the owner of that fingerprint was actually there? Or could that fingerprint have been planted?

Medical doctors use a similar approach. For example, a woman arrives at a doctor with pain in her lower abdomen and she is bleeding vaginally. The doctor asks whether she's pregnant, but the woman emphatically denies it. However, the doctor recognises that these symptoms are probably related to pregnancy, so he performs a pregnancy test. He discovers that his patient is carrying an ectopic pregnancy (a pregnancy in the fallopian tube), which could prove fatal. It later emerges that the woman wasn't ready to acknowledge her condition – the doctor's scepticism saved her life.

In the same way, forensic pathologists should always remain sceptical. They can't even assume that they are dealing with a specific kind of case. For example, if you were called out to a scene where someone was hanging from a beam, and you assumed it was a hanging, you might miss a staged homicide case. Experts call this fallacy of reasoning premature closure. We are supposed to collect all the evidence – then, the results will take shape by themselves.

A story that helps to illustrate this further comes from a death scene where something just did not feel right to me. Two boys, aged twelve and thirteen, had been playing inside a low-cost house in a small informal settlement just outside the city when one of them had apparently committed suicide. When I arrived at the scene, the thirteen-year-old boy recounted the events to me.

'My friend said he was feeling sad and wanted to kill himself,' he said. 'I told my friend not to kill himself but then he said he wanted to stab himself.'

According to the boy he found his friend dead on the living room floor when he walked out of the kitchen area. His friend had a knife in his chest, 'So I pulled the knife out,' the boy continued.

The deceased's body had blood on the front of the shirt and he was lying face-up on the floor. The blood-stained knife was lying next to the body on the right side. The detectives did a thorough examination of the room and the knife was taken as evidence.

I performed the medicolegal post-mortem examination on the boy the following day. What I found surprises me to this day. When I investigated the boy's T-shirt, I noticed that the entrance wound was located overlying the right breast region. I found this odd. Self-inflicted stab wounds to the chest are usually aimed at the heart or precordium. As a side note, most people think that their heart is located on the left side of their chest, but it is actually in the middle-front of the chest, which is why when people try to stab themselves in the heart they often end up puncturing their left lung!

Be that as it may, the entrance wound on the T-shirt looked atypical. Upon removing the skin and muscles on the front chest wall, the wound also looked atypical – and it was atypical when I looked at the wound through the right upper lung too. There was a contusion ring with a diameter of approximately 5 cm. And then I noticed it – a light-calibre projectile located in front of the right scapula bone.

From my investigation of the clothing and the wounds, I

was able to reconstruct what had actually happened. The thirteen-year-old boy had shot the twelve-year-old boy in the right front of the chest. He had then taken a kitchen knife and stuck it into the gunshot entrance wound.

When confronted with our version of events, the thirteen-year-old confessed to his crime. He explained that he had shot his friend by accident when they were playing with their dad's light-calibre weapon. The gun was found at the bottom of one of the dustbins outside the house; he had tried to hide it.

I was astounded at the level of ingenuity and resourcefulness of a thirteen-year-old boy. I could not believe that such a young kid could have devised such a crafty strategy, and it made me fearful of what an adult could do to conceal a murder when given the necessary time and resources.

On a related point, in forensic pathology one should take care not to mistake the unobserved with the unobservable. There are things you cannot see because you don't know what to look for, and there are things you cannot see because they are simply not visible under normal light conditions. Pathology might be staring you in the face, but if you have no experience of it or haven't read about it before, you will probably miss it.

Once, while cutting open the brain of a man who had fallen off a ladder, a piece of mucus-like material, smaller than a baby pea, floated in the cerebrospinal fluid of one of the ventricles. If you've never seen this before, you would miss it, but my colleague realised it was a cysticercus cyst. He had seen one before.

Taenia solium is a cestode parasite, or a tapeworm, which

invades tissue and causes cysticercus infection. The man had accidentally ingested undercooked pork, which contained *Taenia solium* cysticerci, and the route of infection had led these tapeworms to enter his brain. The tapeworms either caused him to have a convulsion or gave rise to sudden raised intracranial pressure, which in turn caused him to fall off the ladder. He may have died due to a head injury, but the reason he fell off the ladder was most likely due to the cysticercus infection.

As mentioned earlier, you often use different light sources to look for pathology. Once, I had been looking at a lung specimen under normal light microscopy. It looked perfectly normal. However, when I looked at the same slide under polarised light, the lung tissue seemed to be full of birefringent 'hot-cross-bun'-shaped foreign material.

What was this stuff?

It turned out to be talcum powder. The deceased was a known recreational drug user, who had used heroine cut with talcum powder. When he had injected the heroine into a vein, the talcum powder had sequestrated in his lungs – just like debris that sequestrates between the reeds of a river system's reedbed.

Something else that can be difficult to identify is Temik (aldicarb) poisoning. Aldicarb is a carbamate insecticide, which is the active substance in the pesticide Temik. Criminals often use food laced with Temik to poison watchdogs, but it has also been used to poison humans. In the gastric contents, Temik granules look exactly like small pepper granules and can easily fool you. Experience is what helps you make the correct diagnosis.

It takes years of blood, sweat and tears to develop mastery of one's field. There are a few tricks of the trade, which newly qualified pathologists are always keen to know. But these gems usually only come with experience and hard work.

Let me share one such secret with you, which concerns hangings. How do you establish whether a hanging is suicidal or homicidal? If you think you would use the height at which they are hanging, the knot used, or the position of the chair on which they stood, you would be wrong.

A crafty murderer may drug a person or subdue him or her with an electronic handheld device before hanging him or her up. A murderer may even fake a suicide note. How, then, does one differentiate between murder and suicide in hanging? The answer took years and years of careful observation by brilliant forensic pathologists from all over the world – and was known before the advent of CT or MRI scans. It is so obvious, yet so invisible to those who did not know what to look for. It has to do with the saliva of the deceased. If someone was alive at the time of the hanging, you will notice a dried rivulet of saliva at the corner of the mouth, diametrically opposite the point of suspension of the noose. To produce saliva, one has to be alive at the time of hanging. If the saliva trail is absent, alarm bells go off; the typical hanging becomes atypical, and homicide should be considered.

Another tip is to look out for hair trapped in the knot of the noose. The typical hanging shouldn't have scalp hair trapped in the knot of the noose because most people want to kill themselves in a way that doesn't hurt. So, if we find hair trapped in the knot of the noose, there is a strong possibility that it is a homicide.

Lead poisoning is another cause of death that can be tricky to spot or observe. It is only after you have seen the so-called blue line in a person's gums that you would suspect lead poisoning. The same goes for the Mees' lines (otherwise known as Aldrich–Mees lines or leukonychia), which are white lines across the fingernails that suggest heavy metal poisoning. The average observer would not notice these lines.

This brings me to a rather difficult ethical question. What are the ethics of diagnosing pathology in a living person whom you do not know, and who is not formally your patient? As a doctor, having taken the modern version of the Hippocratic oath, you may feel it is your duty to tell people what you are noticing. Isn't this why you studied medicine? If someone is sitting next to you on a flight for several hours and you notice multiple small white dots on his forehead (molluscum contagiosum – caused by the pox virus), do you tell him? What would you do if you see a lesion on the back of someone's leg, which clearly looks like a malignant melanoma?

This kind of knowledge and insight into people's behaviour patterns and habits would offend most people, but most doctors are hard-wired to think like this. It is part and parcel of basic medical training. Still, I have discovered – through painful experience – that it is best simply to say, 'Please get that mole checked out by a professional.'

8

Risking life for death

If you want to be a forensic pathologist on the African continent, you have to be prepared for anything. Every day you go to work you are at risk: you never know what may be lurking inside – or outside – a dead body. I have been present when a cocked and loaded gun has fallen out of a victim's trousers, and I have found sharp knives, needles and even screwdrivers on bodies.

There is nothing more terrifying than the silence of a drop of blood. Working in a mortuary, it is impossible to hear the smallest drop of blood splash or drop onto you. Sometimes, one looks at one's notes, or visor, or protective goggles, and there it is – the smallest droplet of blood, which could contain billions, if not trillions, of highly infectious virus particles.

Due to these risks, you need the kind of infrastructure that allows you to investigate fatalities resulting from contagious and/or toxic agents. In other words, is the physical plant sufficiently safe for you to be able to do a good job? Sadly, most autopsy facilities on the continent are in really poor condition. Substantial changes are required, in policies and procedures as well as in the personal protective equipment provided. Glove punctures, for instance, may cause pre-existing hand lesions to be bathed in infectious blood for prolonged periods, without your even feeling it.

All autopsies carry a significant risk of transmitting disease, either by aerosols or through the use of sharp instruments. To prevent exposure, pathologists are now mandated to wear a disposable gown, surgical scrubs, a mask, head protection, eye protection, an apron, sleeve covers, and cut-resistant as well as latex (or rubber) gloves. Unlike surgery on living patients, it is not essential that our gloves and scrubs are sterile. In surgery you want to protect the patient from the surgeon, whereas in forensic pathology you want to protect the pathologist from the deceased.

Infectious risks at an autopsy include HIV, hepatitis and *Mycobacterium tuberculosis*. HIV may be demonstrated in a corpse for up to sixteen and a half days after death. There is a very real possibility of catching HIV from a corpse. South Africa has one of the highest burdens of people living with HIV in the world (7.52 million in 2018). Eastern and sub-Saharan Africa have the highest prevalence of HIV infections: in 2018, there were roughly 37.9 million people living with HIV and 1.7 million new infections.[18]

Almost all my colleagues and co-workers have been on antiretroviral medication due to needle-prick accidents during autopsies at one or other stage of their careers. I have been on antiretrovirals myself several times in my career, due to accidental splashes and cuts. Having said this, at the time of writing I am not aware of any forensic pathologist, locally or internationally, who has seroconverted and become HIV positive due to an injury on duty.

Tuberculosis is a serious and common illness in South Africa, and an autopsy is an exceptionally efficient method of transmitting it from the deceased to those present in the dissection room. The Mantoux test is a test for immunity to tuberculosis. In a study published in 1994 about an outbreak of tuberculosis among medical students at the University of Sydney, eight of thirty-five Mantoux-negative medical students who were exposed to tuberculosis for one hour became infected.[19] The infection risk did not vary with the distance from the autopsy table. Autopsy exposure for as short a time as ten minutes has resulted in transmission of tuberculosis to an observing medical student.[20] Pathologists often have a higher risk of contracting tuberculosis than the clinicians who cared for the patient before death. Even though our patients do not sneeze or cough, they remain infectious. Over the years, I have had two colleagues contract tuberculosis.

I have performed autopsies on some highly contagious cases and only realised what I had been exposed to after the fact. Often, we receive sudden unexpected deaths (known as SUDA, or sudden unexpected deaths in adults), with no history available. Only later, once the special investigations have come back, do we get the results. For example, I have performed at least eight autopsies in my career on meningococcal meningitis cases, all of which seemed to have eluded the clinical surveillance system. In many developed countries, this highly feared disease would probably not even be autopsied.

Meningococcal meningitis is a rare but serious bacterial infection that causes the membranes that cover the brain and spinal cord to become inflamed. Each year, many people die from meningococcal disease, which includes meningitis and septicaemia (blood infection). It usually spreads in dormitories and kills young people. Headache in the morning, dead at night – that is how infectious it is.

The eight contagious cases I had worked on each required a swift, if not highly inconvenient, outbreak response, which entailed tracing and tracking down every contact, every cleaner, every doctor, every nurse and every detective who had come into contact with the deceased. Every single contact with such a case also requires antibiotic prophylaxis.

The best body to work on from an infection point of view is probably a decomposed body (perhaps in the green or black stage of decomposition), because most of the viruses are probably no longer transmissible.

The most feared infectious agents are prions. Prions are proteinaceous infectious particles that lack nucleic acids (they possess neither DNA nor RNA).[21] They are misfolded proteins that characterise several fatal neurodegenerative diseases in animals and humans. It is not known what causes the normal protein to misfold; the abnormal 3D structure is suspected to confer infectious properties.

Prions are hypothesised as the cause of transmissible spongiform encephalopathies, including scrapie in sheep, chronic wasting disease in deer and bovine spongiform encephalopathy – commonly known as mad cow disease – in cattle. In humans, prions have been hypothesised to cause Creutzfeldt–Jakob disease and its variant Gerstmann–Sträussler–Scheinker syndrome, 'fatal familial insomnia' and kuru. A single case of Creutzfeldt–Jakob disease has been reported in a laboratory technician whose work included handling formalin-fixed brains.[22] There is currently no known effective treatment for prion disease. Note that prions are not inactivated by formalin, and retain transmissibility in paraffin blocks. An autopsy on a suspected prion-infected body is therefore the realm of the super specialist. Personally, I wouldn't perform an autopsy on a prion case.

The problem in Africa is that we often have no history when a body is admitted to the mortuary. For instance, when a person is found dead in an informal settlement, we often do not know their nationality, identity or medical history.

I once conducted the autopsy on a woman who had died in her apartment in the city centre. Upon opening her up, it looked like she was infected with the dreaded Ebola, a viral haemorrhagic fever, as all her organs appeared haemorrhagic. Even her omentum had haemorrhagic petechiae (blood spots) on it. This required us to institute quarantine and emergency procedures immediately. After rapid and thorough investigation, it turned out she was an HIV-positive patient with systemic herpes infection. It turns out that, when these two illnesses are combined, it looks exactly like a haemorrhagic fever virus at autopsy.

Health and safety at autopsy is critically important. A high-risk autopsy can be defined as 'post-mortem examination of a deceased person who has had, or is likely to have had, a serious infectious disease that can be transmitted to those present at the autopsy, thereby causing them serious illness and/or premature death'.[23]

In the wake of the COVID-19 pandemic, the high-risk autopsy has never been riskier. Pathogens may be acquired by inhalation (of aerosols), ingestion, direct inoculation, entry through pre-existing breaks in the skin, and through the mucous membranes of the eyes, nose and mouth. Any procedure may result in infection through one of these routes.[24] In the UK, autopsies on Hazard Group 4 pathogens (for example, the viral haemorrhagic fevers) should be performed only when absolutely necessary.[25]

Regarding COVID-19, there are two main scenarios for forensic pathologists. The first, as mentioned earlier, involves a SUDA with no available history. For example, someone is found dead in their residence and has no known history. After a thorough autopsy, it turns out that the person died from a highly infectious disease such as COVID-19. The second involves, for example, someone with a COVID-19 infection who dies an unnatural death, homicide, suicide or accident. In either scenario, the forensic pathologist is at high risk. The answer, therefore, is to treat all forensic deaths as highly infectious. And yes, it is by the grace of God that we enter the mortuary every day. Extreme precautions and protocols are therefore necessary to preserve the safety of the health workers involved in the autopsy procedure of suspected COVID-19 cases.

In addition to infectious diseases, pathologists also face other dangers in the mortuary. The first danger is toxic agents. The most common toxic agent to which forensic pathologists are exposed is formaldehyde, which is used to preserve tissues. Formaldehyde is extremely volatile and causes an array of symptoms, including irritation of the eyes, mucous membranes and skin.[26] Formaldehyde can also cause atopy and hypersensitivity.[27] You should not be able to smell it. If you can, it generally means that you are inhaling a concentration that exceeds the occupational standard. Formaldehyde has been rumoured to cause cancers, specifically cancers of the lung.[28]

Forensic pathologists and their technicians are sometimes exposed to cyanide when performing autopsies on persons who have died after ingesting this substance.[29] Although cyanide can volatilise from autopsy tissues, the major risk to autopsy personnel occurs when the stomach is opened. In the acid gastric environment, cyanide salts are converted to highly volatile hydrocyanic acid. Unless the stomach is opened in a totally exhausted biosafety cabinet or chemical fume hood, forensic practitioners risk inhaling potentially toxic concentrations of this gas.

I have also worked on victims who had been exposed to organophosphate pesticides, such as malathion, parathion and carbamates.[30] These substances may cause toxicity as a consequence of inhalation, ingestion, or dermal absorption. Exposure to gastric contents and clothing containing or contaminated with organophosphate pesticides can be dangerous. In South Africa, organophosphates usually present in the form of aldicarb poisoning. At autopsy, you find multiple small grey-black granules admixed within the gastric contents. Aldicarb is known locally as a 'two-step' death (because if you ingest it orally, which is considered the first step, it kills you in the second step). It is also known locally as *halephirimi*.

Nerve gas agents like tabun, sarin, VX and soman are organophosphate compounds that are used in chemical warfare and bioterrorism. These agents can slowly penetrate heavy rubber gloves and aprons, and be absorbed through the skin.[31]

The best way to decontaminate a body, especially in under-resourced environments, is with copious amounts of running water. I call it the 'green water snake method' – the good old-fashioned green hosepipe remains the gold standard for decontaminating any dead body in Africa.

The second danger is radiation. Autopsy workers may at times be exposed to radioactive material in a body from diagnostic or therapeutic procedures.[32] The extent of radiation exposure is dependent on the dose administered to the patient, the type of radiation emitted, the radionuclide, the exposure time, and the shielding or protection used by the forensic pathologist. A pathologist who performed an autopsy without precautions on an individual who had undergone a gallium-67 scan received an excessive radiation exposure.[33] While radiation experts might be scarce in developing countries, a radiation safety expert should ideally always be consulted before the autopsy to evaluate potential exposure.

The third danger is electronic devices. Implantable cardioverter defibrillators are sometimes used to treat tachyarrhythmias of the heart. Prosectors and forensic pathologists who manipulate these devices or cut the leads may sustain an electrical discharge of 25–40 joules.[34] We might not always know that a defibrillator is present in a body before the autopsy. Some manufacturing companies have representatives available to assist with the deactivation of these devices, but finding such a representative in rural Africa may prove challenging.

The fourth danger is mechanical risks. As mentioned earlier, there are cases on record of bombs being hidden in the bodies of corpses, especially during times of war. There have also been cases of dangerous objects like weapons being hidden on bodies; a loaded gun may fall from the body and discharge its projectile.

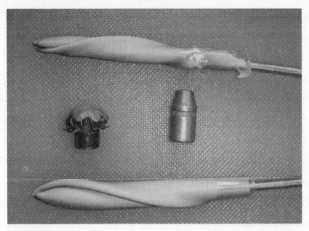

The bullet on the left shows the super sharp petals of a deformed projectile. Rubber-tipped forceps (above and below the bullets) are used to remove such projectiles from a body. *Photo: S Rossouw*

I am aware of a case of a victim being shot with a so-called black talon projectile, which is now known as a ranger projectile. The front of the black talon projectile 'mushrooms', with the sharp edges looking like the petals of a flower. This lethal projectile may easily penetrate even the sturdiest of gloves; you have to be exceptionally cautious when removing these projectiles from a body, or when working inside a body cavity, as they can rip and cut through the gloves. You can easily become infected with the corpse's blood.

The average person will, in their lifetime, perhaps see one or two dead bodies. They might discover the body of a loved one, or see a pedestrian killed on the side of the road while driving past.

Forensic pathologists, however, are constantly exposed to death and dying. After all, in busy centres we work with about twenty to thirty corpses per day; a normal day for a forensic pathologist is a totally abnormal one for any other person.

This brings me to another risk that forensic pathologists face: the psychological impact of doing your job. For one, you may become desensitised to death and dying. For another, we witness things to which most people never have to be exposed, and we have to develop the skills to deal with this. There are death scenes that will forever be etched in my mind. As they say, we don't remember what we want to remember; we remember what we can't forget.

A scene I find particularly hard to forget was when a deranged shooter ran from building to building in the centre of one of our main cities, firing at people. The entire block was the death scene. I had to walk through the scene with ballistics detectives who were showing me how and where the shots were fired, and basically recreating the scene.

This was important from a forensic pathology point of view because I needed to understand the direction from which the shots were fired, whether there were intermediate targets present, etc. It was surreal the way the shooter had jumped and moved from building to building, all the while shooting and killing people. Of course, what must have taken minutes to induce took several days to reconstruct and investigate.

In an action movie, there can be multiple scenes of shooters firing many projectiles and shooting multiple people. Now imagine, for a moment, actually performing the forensics on that gun sequence. Imagine trying to recreate, step by step, the angles and the range of fire of every single gunshot. Imagine investigating the scene and the dead bodies. Then, imagine having to collate all your data in 3D. This is an incredibly labour-intensive and exhausting exercise if done correctly.

There have also been unusual death scenes where we almost risked our lives for someone else's death. At times, we have to go into really unsafe neighbourhoods and ganglands to retrieve bodies. Once, we had to collect a body from an apartment. The lifts in the building did not work, and there were no hoists to lower the body. Hoists are considered a luxury item in developing countries, so manual labour is all we had. This meant that the body had to be carried down multiple flights of stairs. Needless to say, we had to be quite fit to perform this laborious task – especially since the body weighed over 120 kg. We also had to contend with the spectator value it created. People emerged from their flats and apartments and gaped at us, or stared out of windows, some with curlers in their hair.

I often ask my colleagues which death scenes are the toughest they have witnessed. A colleague once attended a death scene on a highway that spanned over a kilometre. It was a single-pedestrian vehicle accident; a pedestrian had been hit by a car that was driving very, very fast. According to my colleague, he and his team walked that entire length of road searching for fragments of the dead pedestrian. The accident had happened in the early-morning hours of a freezing winter's day. He said it was an incredibly eerie feeling, walking along that lonely stretch of highway with the occasional car or truck zooming past. When he eventually found the decapitated head of the deceased and walked back to his vehicle with it in the mist, it felt to him like he was in some strange zombie movie.

Note that as forensic pathologists we never perform autopsies on friends, relatives, or anyone close to us. If a forensic pathologist from one city dies, the protocol is that a forensic pathologist colleague who does not know that individual well should perform the autopsy. This is obviously difficult: all of us who work in a certain region know one another. So, it might even require flying a forensic pathologist in from somewhere else in the country – or the world.

Over the years, I have had many friends and colleagues end up at the mortuary. This has been very hard for me.

I am often asked whether I don't get depressed from seeing so much death and dying. In the USA, medical examiners may perform no more than 250 autopsies per year according to the current standards of the National Association of Medical Examiners (if they exceed this number, the mortuary loses its accreditation). South African forensic pathologists perform on average 250 to 500 autopsies per year. We only had 53 to 56 board-certified and practising forensic pathologists at the time of writing.

Imagine waking up, going to work and having to deal with a beheading case, a multiple gunshot wound case and a multiple stab wound case (with associated rape). Now imagine doing this day after day. A normal, low-key day in the life of an African forensic pathologist is probably beyond comprehension to the layperson.

It is definitely a calling of sorts. Some of us seem to treat the dead better than we treat ourselves.

Due to the numbers of dead, we have had to 'industrialise' the autopsy, so to speak, to prevent us from burning out. This system is based on the saying that many hands make light work. The irony is that, if you work with it every day, there is a certain tedium to death and dying.

It is easy to become desensitised when exposed to this magnitude of death and dying; however, forensic pathologists have the scientific background to look beyond the emotions and focus on the science when we see a dead human body. This is why I am often quite concerned when rookie police officers see their first dead body: they do not have the same scientific background as pathologists do. It really has to be a calling for them, too.

If you are properly trained, however, I believe you will be able to manage most situations and not suffer post-traumatic stress disorder. In fact, most of the forensic pathology professionals I know are extremely positive and optimistic people. Perhaps all the exposure to death and dying has woken them up to life.

We have all processed scenes and conducted examinations that have taken their toll on our collective psyche. However, doing this is also incredibly rewarding. Forensic pathologists are part of a group of professionals who document atrocities and give closure to victims' next of kin. The critical evidence we collect is used to bring perpetrators to justice; we also help exonerate the innocent.

For this reason, I would do this all again in a heartbeat.

9

Ways of dying, part I

There are many ways to die. As forensic pathologists, it is our job to investigate the cause of death. From transport-related deaths and poisoning deaths to torture and freak accidents, we see it all. As mentioned earlier, some of us even have extensive international experience in investigating war crimes, high-profile assassination cases, mass disasters and armed conflict scenarios.

There are many ways in which life's candle may be snuffed out. The Grim Reaper works 24/7 and takes no vacations – death seems to lurk behind every tree and every bush. The randomness and senseless of death tends to make you somewhat philosophical. If you work in this field, you understand that statistics are at play all the time. If you were to take a hundred people, randomly, and follow their lives for an unspecified period, a certain percentage will develop cancer, a number of them will commit suicide, some will be murdered; others will die from natural causes, or in an accident.

Looking at other parameters, a certain percentage will become a boss, others will become employees and some will lose their jobs; many will get married and have kids, while others will remain single; many will travel, but others will not; a certain number will be very religious, and others will lose all faith; some people will find their purpose in life, and others never.

Statistics can be looked at in various ways. The chances of winning the UK National Lottery are 1 in 13 983 816. However, statistically this is incorrect: from your personal point of view, the real statistical chances of winning the UK Lottery are 50 per cent – either you win, or you lose!

The statistics of unnatural death should be viewed in the same way. From your personal point of view, you have a 50 per cent chance of an unnatural death. Either it will happen to you, or it will not.

A mother and a child stop at a convenience store to buy milk. A stray bullet from a nearby shooting penetrates both mother and child, and kills both instantaneously. A man gets out of his car to change a tyre. A speeding car hits him as he gets out of his vehicle, killing him immediately. I have seen this happen more than once. Then there was the case of the man walking on the side of the road with his girlfriend when a wheel came off a car, flew through the air, and fatally hit him on the head from behind.

So many variables play a role in the creation of an accident. For example, if you accidentally trip over a cord on the floor in your house, someone must have left the cord there in the first place; you must have been sufficiently distracted not to see the cord; and the timing of you and the cord being there at that specific time must coincide. Accidents do not happen just randomly – an accident is a perfect storm of multiple events that all come together to create the moment of the accident.

I have also dealt with no fewer than three instances of a groom-to-be dying at his own bachelor party. One drowned, one caught fire while trying to light a braai with petrol, and the third died of alcohol poisoning. I have even had a case of a groom dying on his wedding night. While he was with his beautiful bride in their bedroom, criminals entered the room and mugged them. He was tragically shot in the ensuing scuffle, and died.

The randomness and senselessness of it all boggles my mind. It leaves me wondering: is there any lesson or message in such tragic, unnatural deaths? Speaking of randomness, I have seen a case of a man being shot multiple times by gang members, and having an expert surgeon save his life. And I have seen a victim who sustained a minor blow to the head during a common pub brawl, and died immediately. The pub victim had an eggshell skull, which means that his skull was thinner than normal.

The gun-wielding gangsters received lesser sentences in court than the man who punched the guy in the pub. It is still hard for me to believe that shooters would be punished less harshly than a fist-fighter. If the surgeon hadn't saved the gunshot victim's life, the gangsters would probably have received harsher sentences.

In the first chapter, I described some of the quickest and most painless ways to die. I explained that a nuclear death, a lightning death, or jumping into an active volcano would probably bring the quickest death, and that beheading by guillotine would be a relatively slow death by comparison.

I have witnessed some really slow and painful deaths in my

career. For some, life is too long; for others it is too short. Some of these slow deaths still haunt me.

One of the most tragic and slowest deaths I have seen was caused by a snoek bone. The snoek, *Thyrsites atun*, is a long, thin species of mackerel found in the seas of the southern hemisphere. Snoek is a classic South African delicacy. A middle-aged woman accidentally swallowed a snoek bone, which perforated her small intestine. She spent a year in hospital because the perforation caused a fistula (an abnormal passage between two hollow or tubular organs). She ended up developing a chronic peritonitis (an infection of the abdomen). The year she spent in the ward involved multiple surgeries to try to clear up the infection. Eventually, after a year of agony, anger and depression, she succumbed to sepsis.

One of the strangest and quickest deaths I have had to investigate involved white socks. A middle-aged man who was wearing only white socks and a pair of white underpants had gone into his kitchen and apparently slipped on the smooth floor. He cracked his skull and died on the spot. After a thorough scene reconstruction and autopsy, the precipitating cause of death was, most likely, the slippery floor and the socks.

There is a condition in forensic pathology known as INCA, or instantaneous neurogenic cardiac arrest, which presents another quick way to die. INCA describes the immediate and complete cessation of myocardial activity caused by a neural stimulus. This is a very strange and rare condition, but cases of INCA are of major medicolegal importance.[35]

Here are a few examples of INCA-related deaths:[36]

- A soldier playfully tweaked his girlfriend's neck on the dance floor. The next moment, she dropped dead. Pressure changes in the carotid artery may interfere with a person's baroreceptors.[37] A similar case occurred where a grandmother kissed her grandchild and applied pressure to the child's neck. The child died instantly.

- Compression of the neck (caused, for example, by a high, stiff collar that exerts pressure on the carotid sinus when one turns one's head, a tie suddenly constricted around the neck, or even pressure during intense love-making). There is a case on record of so-called Eagle syndrome (prolonged stylohyoid processes), in which sudden death was caused by merely turning the head.[38]

- Application of extreme blunt force to the stomach (such as in a belly flop into water), the solar plexus or pit of the stomach, the philtrum of the lip, the inner aspect of the knee, or the genitalia (notably the testes) may cause INCA.

- Sudden cold water to the male external genitalia may also cause instantaneous neurogenic cardiac arrest. For example, a man may be drinking alcohol in the warm sun and then run into the cold ocean water, and suddenly die. This cold shock response is known as hydrocution.

- In the oculocardiac reflex, or so-called diving reflex, pressure on the eyeballs may slow the heart due to parasympathetic effect. Compression of the eyeballs produces reflex bradycardia, which is a slowing of the rhythm of the heart.

- The glottis is highly sensitive. Stimulation of the nasopharynx area (the upper part of your throat, behind the nose) by a sudden gush of cold water into this area may cause an INCA-related death. Foreign objects, such as a food bolus, lodged in the pharynx may cause a 'café coronary death', which is not the same as choking.

- Sudden dilatation of the uterine cervix, especially during illicit abortion, or of the anal sphincter during anal rape may have a similar effect.

While no specific post-mortem signs are found in INCA cases, the post-mortem diagnosis of 'death due to INCA' is not used as a general stopgap whenever the cause of death cannot be established. The facial features at death in INCA are typically pale, composed or peaceful. It remains a strange phenomenon that we, as humans, have such a cut-off switch, which only gets stimulated under very specific circumstances.

People ask me whether one can die from fear or emotional stress. Rigorous proof that someone has dropped dead of fright is currently inaccessible to the pathologist, and will probably remain so.[39] There is, however, no doubt that some people are more prone to developing cardiac arrhythmias than others. Some people may have underlying ischaemic heart disease. Maybe the hearts of such people are primed to fibrillate when circulating catecholamines (for example, adrenaline) are unusually high, as in apprehension of sudden attack. Sudden mental shock may probably cause an INCA, for instance from receiving very upsetting news, which may stimulate the parasympathetic nervous system; anxiety and pain may stimulate the sympathetic nervous system. Deaths in such circumstances are probably physiological.

A much more common cause of death in South Africa is projectiles (bullets). Finding and extracting projectiles from a human body is a really labour-intensive task. The most difficult places from which to remove projectiles during autopsy are from the facial sinuses, the hip bones and the vertebral column. The mastoid bone behind the ear is also a particularly difficult region.

These areas are hard to reach – and, of course, it is important for us to remove the projectiles without damaging the evidence on the projectile or causing further cosmetic damage to the body. For example, removing a projectile from a facial sinus without damaging the cosmetic features of the face can be very tricky.

Over the years, I've seen a range of deadly projectiles. While military projectiles are designed according to particular specifications, civilian projectiles are designed according to a completely different set of rules. The military-minded weapon and projectile maker designs projectiles that perforate the human body and armour, and cause maximum fatalities with minimal casualties. In other words, the bullets should go right through the body, killing the person immediately and not dumping any of the projectile's energy inside the body.

The civilian weapon and projectile maker, on the other hand, does not want to kill, but rather to injure the criminal who tries to attack or rob the user of the weapon. So, the idea is for the bullet to dump all its energy inside the criminal, and hurt, but not kill, the criminal – otherwise, the civilian would be up for murder or manslaughter. This is why civilian projectile designers design bullets with weird and wonderful shapes and characteristics. There are bullets with flat tops, hollow points or petal-like openings on the projectile fronts. As paradoxical as it sounds, civilians want the bullet to stop and expand within their victims, dumping all their energy but not necessarily killing the victim. In other words, they only want to hurt the criminal – not kill the criminal.

For this reason, civilian projectiles scare me the most. I have seen shotgun cartridges filled with seeds, salt, sand and even cyanide powder. People come up with all sorts of projectiles in the comfort of their own homes.

In forensics, ballistics is a super speciality. There are three main fields: weapon ballistics, flight ballistics and terminal ballistics. The weapon ballistics specialist is the expert on the weapon itself, whereas the flight ballistics specialist is the expert on the dynamics of the projectile flying through the air. The terminal ballistics specialist is the expert on the effects of the projectile on the body. The forensic pathologist deals chiefly with terminal ballistics.

Forensic analysts require the bullet to perform ballistics tests. Every time a bullet leaves the barrel of a gun, the barrel and the gun leave a 'fingerprint' on that specific bullet, which may link it forensically to that specific weapon. This is why it is so very important for us to find projectiles on crime scenes or in dead bodies. The projectile may be linked to the gun, by means of Locard's principle.

There is a very strange phenomenon in forensics called 'vanishing projectile syndrome': one gunshot entrance wound to the body is detected, but no projectile can be found in the body, despite a thorough examination. We approach this puzzle as follows. First, we ask 'anomaly-seeking' questions. Perhaps the gunshot entrance wound was not an *ipso facto* gunshot entrance wound at all. It may, for example, have been a crossbow arrow injury, and the person who fired the bow may have removed the crossbow arrow from the wound. The skin entrance wound from a crossbow arrow looks almost exactly like that of a gunshot entrance wound.

A projectile could also ricochet out of the wound. For example, it could hit a bone and then 'bounce' back out of the wound. Or the projectile could travel into the body and out through an orifice (mouth, ear, nostril or vagina). When we examine the body of such a gunshot wound victim, we will find no projectiles.

We also take atypical wound factors into account. For example, a tangential gunshot wound may give the impression of a gunshot entrance wound, but the projectile merely skimmed the surface of the body. In such cases, no projectile will be found within the body. If a projectile passes tangentially through the underside of a breast, the corner of an armpit or between the base of the fingers of a hand, it may appear to be an atypical gunshot entrance wound, whereas it is actually a tangential gunshot wound through an unusually contoured part of the body. No projectile will be found within the body in such cases.

A bullet could also embolise within the body. For example, a bullet fired into the aorta may travel down the lumen of a large artery, such as the aorta, and embolise within one of the limbs of the victim, making discovery of the projectile very difficult.

A bullet can also be removed by the suspect (in rare cases) or the surgeon (more common). To the uninitiated, many a surgical drain that has been removed in the emergency room looks almost exactly like a gunshot wound – but no projectile will be found in the body of such cases, of course.

In one case, I noticed on X-ray what I thought was a malformed projectile in the face of the deceased. It looked as if the bullet was lodged deep within the nasal cavity. After a lengthy examination, the bullet turned out to be a piece of gauze, which is commonly used by ENT specialists. This crumpled-up piece of gauze really fooled me. The gauze was impregnated with a bismuth subnitrate, iodoform and paraffin paste, which is radio-opaque.

Another unique case showed a perforating gunshot wound through the right foot, and another through the right lower leg, the right upper leg and also through the right upper arm and right forearm. To summarise, in total there were ten gunshot wounds on the body.

But, believe it or not, the guy had been shot only once. He had been climbing over a wall when he had been shot. The projectile had entered his foot and then exited it before entering his lower leg and exiting it. Next, it re-entered his upper leg and exited it, after which it entered his upper arm. It then exited the upper arm, re-entered his forearm and exited his forearm.

When the body was lying flat on the autopsy table in the anatomical position, it appeared to have been shot multiple times. But all the wounds lined up in a neat pattern. This is why one should always try to think three-dimensionally and in slow motion when reconstructing gunshot wound cases.

On X-ray examination, the projectile may appear to be within the body itself, but we have had incidents of projectiles being trapped between the clothing and the body. When you undress the body, the projectile may fall out. It is always surprising when a projectile falls out of a deceased's clothing on the autopsy table.

Finding a bullet is often like finding a needle in a haystack. For instance, digging a bullet out of the soil in a garden can be tedious and will require a metal detector.

Gunshot wound fatalities that happen in the victim's bed – whether they are suicidal, accidental, or homicidal – are really difficult to investigate, and hard work. The public rarely appreciates this from a forensic-investigative and cleaning-up point of view. Do you have any idea how hard it is to find and remove a bullet that is trapped inside a mattress? There are layers upon layers of material and sponge and springs. It is also near impossible to remove blood stains from a mattress. You can clean the surface layers, but the inner layers will forever remain a silent witnesses to what happened.

It is also tough to dig a projectile out of a concrete wall, a wooden wall, a dry wall, or a ceiling.

We also encounter cases of so-called mob assault. Mob assault or vigilante homicide is a form a community assault. The typical mob assault involves a group of people from a specific community who attack an individual they believe has done something wrong. Interestingly, the attacks I have seen have mostly been on men. The pathology of trauma of mob assault cases is fascinating, as the exact cause of death is rarely clear.

The mode of mob assault has changed over the years. A particularly brutal form of mob assaults we encountered in the past was necklacing. As mentioned earlier, this entails placing a rubber tyre filled with petrol around a victim's chest and arms, and setting it alight. Nowadays, we are seeing a lot of mob assault cases that are due to multiple directed blunt force trauma (beating with sticks and stones). The attackers usually use flexible sticks, such as sjamboks, but sometimes they also use rigid sticks. Use of the sjambok explains why our victims are often covered with so-called tramline injuries.

The attackers may also use stones. This is stoning in the biblical sense. The pathology of stoning injuries is very specific and can fool even the most experienced of pathologists. Stoning does not result in circular bruises all over the body, as one would expect. It may cause strange injuries indeed. Often, stoning victims have unusual abrasions, lacerations and contusions over their bodies.

In some mob assault cases, the attackers throw an accelerant, such as petrol or paraffin, over the genitals as a *coup de grâce*. We often see burn wounds on mob assault victims.

Now, here is the fascinating thing: when we dissect these mob assault bodies at autopsy, the internal organs show almost no injuries. One would expect to find skull fractures, or broken ribs, or a subdural haematoma of the brain or an extradural haematoma of the head – yet, remarkably, the internal organs are in pristine condition. So, why do these people die? This remains one of the greatest mysteries in modern forensics. Currently, we have five theories of the cause of death in such instances:

- The victims bleed to death due to blood loss under their skin. We think that the extreme blunt force trauma suffered by these victims causes them to bleed subcutaneously to the extent that they lose up to three litres of blood – perhaps more.
- The victims have raised potassium levels (hyperkalaemia) due to the red blood cells that rupture during severe external blunt force trauma. We suspect that such raised potassium levels can affect the heart, causing an arrhythmia.

- The victim's adrenaline and noradrenaline levels become so high due to the dynamic events of the mob assault that they affect the heart, causing an arrhythmia and death.
- The victims die from positional asphyxia when they are placed in a position that compromises their normal breathing.
- The victims may suffer an INCA due to extreme emotion or pain, which causes sympathetic nervous system overload and death.

It is very hard to prosecute such mobs and bring them to justice, unless we find a spot of blood from one of the attackers on the clothing of the victim, or vice versa. Unless, of course, the assault is filmed, which happens surprisingly often these days since nearly everyone has a mobile phone with a camera.

Yet another cause of death that South African forensic pathologists often encounter is alcohol. People really love alcohol, in good times and in bad times – at all times, in fact.

A description of the mode of action of alcohol on the human body – how alcohol gets absorbed by the human body, and how it is eliminated – is beyond the scope of this book. Suffice to say that the clinical examination of a person under the influence of alcohol should be directed towards ascertaining whether the person's faculties are impaired.

At the same time, an attempt should be made to determine whether impairment of function is wholly due to alcohol, or due to drugs, other substances, trauma, physical or mental disorder or disease. For example, a person may look drunk when in fact he or she has a head injury. I once investigated a case where everyone thought the deceased was drunk, but it turned out that the cause of death was a subdural haematoma of the brain due to blunt force head trauma.

In another case, it was thought that the deceased had died because he had been hit on the head, but it turned out that he had died from alcohol poisoning.

Alcohol can kill you, either acutely (quickly) or chronically (slowly). An example of an acute death due to alcohol was the groom-to-be who died from alcohol poisoning at his bachelor party. I have also seen people commit suicide by drinking whole bottles of cane, gin or whiskey. Severe alcoholism can cause Korsakoff psychosis, which could cause memory deficits, confusion and behavioural changes. Delirium tremens is a rapid onset of confusion usually caused by withdrawal from alcohol. When it occurs, it is often approximately three days into the withdrawal and typically lasts for two to three days. People have died from Korsakoff psychosis and delirium tremens.

In acute alcohol poisoning, death occurs at blood alcohol concentrations of over 0.35 grams per 100 millilitres. Stupor or coma or danger from aspirating vomit occurs at blood alcohol concentrations of between 0.30 and 0.35 grams per 100 millilitres.

With regard to chronic effects, I have seen people die from cirrhosis (scarring) of the liver, pancreatitis and Wernicke's encephalopathy (a type of neurological condition caused by thiamine deficiency, which primarily affects the peripheral and central nervous systems). Alcohol can affect almost every organ system in your body, from the brain to the eyes and the skin.

It is for these reasons that one should drink in moderation, or not at all.

It always surprises me how many of our unnatural deaths have alcohol on board at the time of death. Alcohol is without a doubt one of South Africa's most abused substances.

10
Ways of dying, part II

In my line of work, I get to see the results of many different kinds of addictions. Some people are addicted to food, especially carbohydrates and sugar. Others are addicted to alcohol, smoking, sex or adrenaline.

You can spot the signs of addiction both internally and externally if you look closely enough. For instance, the thickness of the anterior abdominal fat wall or the amount of fat around the kidneys gives one a relatively good idea of carbohydrate intake. The pericardial and the epicardial fat content also reveals a lot about a person's eating habits.

I can usually also tell whether a person was a smoker when they lie on my autopsy table. I simply have to look at their skin. Smoking destroys the enzyme elastase, and the connective tissue loses its elasticity. The face of a smoker is usually wrinkled; even the skin on the dorsal aspects of the smoker's hands loses its elasticity.

And then there are drugs.

Nyaope is one of the cheapest, widespread, most dangerous and highly addictive drugs in the country. Nyaope users inject themselves with the drug and then draw their own blood and pass the syringe to others who hope to get a high. This is called bluetoothing. Obviously, this is a dangerous and foolish practice. You have approximately five litres of blood in your body. When you inject a drug into your body, it gets tremendously diluted and passes through your liver, which acts like a filter. It is virtually impossible to get high from someone else's drugged blood.

The only thing that will happen is a so-called blood transfusion reaction (one person's blood will react with the other person's blood) and there will be a great chance of contracting HIV, hepatitis C, or some other nasty infection.

I am intrigued by how drugs get into the country and onto the streets. Drug cartels are very sophisticated and many use people as mules to transport drugs across borders. These mules are entirely expendable to the cartels. Drugs are typically put into condoms, balloons, or the finger-ends of latex gloves. These 'bullets' are then placed in the mule's vagina, rectum, mouth, ear, nose, or even foreskin. If swallowed, the mules take loperamide (Immodium) to decrease gut motility. Mules are also referred to as body packers or stuffers. I am aware of cases in which as much as a kilogram of cocaine was swallowed. The packages are typically 25 mm × 15 mm containers. At the journey's end, the mule takes laxatives in order to pass the packages.

The bullets or drug packages often leak, which may cause overdosing and death. If they suspect they are about to be arrested, the mules can quickly swallow the drugs, even though they may not be that well wrapped. If you are flying overseas and a fellow passenger suddenly gets up, looking sweaty and like they are burning up with fever, it could be from a ruptured drug package.

There are cases on record of foreign nationals who are found dead in a hotel close to an airport or train station. The death scene is typical; there are laxatives nearby, and the deceased might be covered with wet towels or there could be ice strewn about. Some have also been found sitting on a chair, with an electric fan or air conditioner blasting them. If a drug package bursts inside the mule's gastrointestinal tract, the extreme overdose of cocaine causes very high temperatures.

If they swallowed heroin, there may be foaming around the face. There are even reported cases of a body having been cut open by the drug cartels to retrieve the drugs.

The sophisticated cartels dissolve the drugs with substances that have the same radiodensity of human stools. This makes detection of these drugs almost impossible on normal X-ray. CT scanning or barium contrast studies are required to identify these packages.

Medical management of such cases remains controversial. Some surgeons let the drugs pass through the gastrointestinal tract, and others cut them out. Obviously, each specific drug mule case will have to be managed individually.

It astounds and saddens me to see how many young women end up as prostitutes on the streets. I have so often heard different versions of the story: a young small-town woman arrives in a big city. She goes to a club where she meets a woman of her age. This woman offers her a pill, and tells her she shouldn't worry about it, it's not a drug and that it will simply let her have a good time. The pill would be called Mary Jane, E or Liquid Quaalude, for example. The woman reluctantly accepts the pill and has a great time.

The next week, she returns to the club and finds her friend.

Once again, she has her magic pill and has a good time. The third time she meets her friend and asks for the magic pill, the friend introduces the woman to her supplier – typically a big guy working for a drug cartel. He pulls out a little black book and proceeds to tell her that she owes him money. He might also tell her that he knows the name of her parents and siblings, and where they live. He might even tell her the name of her pet dog or cat.

Within weeks, the innocent woman is trapped by the cartel. The magic pill was cocaine or an amphetamine, or maybe even heroine, which is *highly* addictive. No matter who you are, or how strong you think you are, you *will* become addicted. From the autopsy table, it is often difficult to get the full backstory. But every now and again, it filters through.

Another way in which a large number of South Africans die annually is transport related. I have seen many horrific road traffic fatalities.

Many of the vehicles on Southern African roads are not roadworthy. There are cases on record of unroadworthy cars that have leaked exhaust fumes into the cabin of the vehicle itself while it was being driven, and of all the occupants being overcome by carbon monoxide gas.

In South Africa and on the rest of the continent, cattle and goats tend to roam free in certain parts. Every now and again, we have to perform the autopsy on a driver who accidentally drove into a cow, a goat or a donkey. There have also been cases of people hitting hippopotami, kudu and impala. Animals on the road aside, it can be especially dangerous driving late at night in South Africa because drunk drivers tend to be on the road in the early hours of the morning.

Some people should simply not be allowed behind a steering wheel because they do not have enough confidence or skill to drive a car. Others are too impatient and reckless, and drive too fast, risking both pedestrians and other drivers. Having these two types of drivers share our roads is a recipe for disaster. Maybe the future of transport is driverless, electric cars that run on artificial intelligence.

The bulk of our workload in terms of transport-related deaths involves pedestrian vehicle accidents, however. The first ever pedestrian vehicle accident victim in the world was a British woman called Bridget Driscoll, who died on 17 August 1896 when she was struck by a car belonging to the Anglo-French Motor Carriage Company that was being used to give demonstration rides.

One witness described the car as travelling at 'a reckless pace, in fact, like a fire engine'. Although the car's maximum speed was 8 miles per hour (13 km/h), it had been limited deliberately to 4 miles per hour (6.4 km/h). The accident happened just a few weeks after a new Act of Parliament had increased the speed limit for cars to 14 miles per hour (23 km/h), from 2 miles per hour in towns and 4 miles per hour in the countryside. The jury returned a verdict of accidental death and the coroner said he hoped 'such a thing would never happen again'.

In forensics, we get high-velocity pedestrian vehicle accidents, where people are hit by vehicles on highways travelling at great speeds (60–100 km/h), and low-velocity pedestrian vehicle accidents, where people are hit by cars in the suburbs, travelling at relatively slower speeds (20–60 km/h).[40] The difference in pathology of trauma between the two cases is remarkable. The high-velocity pedestrian accident victims are grossly disfigured. The lower-velocity pedestrian vehicle accident victims tend to be more intact, with chiefly head and lower limb injuries.

Every now and again, we get hit-and-run pedestrian vehicle accidents. We then have to try to find the car. Fortunately, the pedestrian and the car leave traces of themselves on each other (according to Locard's principle, mentioned earlier). We might find glass or paint on the deceased pedestrian's body or clothes, or blood, clothing, or hair on the offending vehicle.

There is a case on record of a motor vehicle accident victim who was lying on a gurney after having sustained minor injuries in the accident. Minutes later, he was dead. He had only minor abrasions, according to the ambulance personnel. It was quite a mystery. The body was sent for a medicolegal autopsy, and it was established that he died from carbon monoxide poisoning from the ambulance's exhaust fumes. He had been placed relatively close to the exhaust pipe of the ambulance while the paramedics attended to the other occupants of the vehicle. Carbon monoxide binds 250 times more strongly to haemoglobin than oxygen; the cause of death, then, had little to do with the initial motor vehicle accident, and everything to do with the carbon monoxide-rich exhaust fumes from the ambulance.

I have also seen plenty of taxi-related deaths over the years. By law, taxis are allowed to accommodate only fifteen passengers, but at times they take on more; they are often not roadworthy, and some taxi drivers may have fake driver's licences. From time to time, we perform autopsies on multiple people who died in a taxi accident.

Then there are the deaths caused by taxi violence. Often, a taxi boss will hire youngsters to kill the competition. This is when we end up having to perform an autopsy on a bullet-ridden rival taxi boss. These are not always easy cases to investigate, because there are usually multiple gunshot wounds, from multiple different ranges and directions. To make the investigation even more challenging, the bullet entrance wounds are often atypical (because the victims have been shot through a vehicle's doors and windows). Multiple secondary projectile fragments enter the bodies, which are often tough to locate.

Then there are people who become so depressed that they decide to take their own life. Every forty seconds, a suicide takes place somewhere on the globe – there are about 800 000 suicides a year. Countries with high suicide rates include Belarus, Lithuania, Kazakhstan, Russia and Japan; countries with low suicide rates are Jordan, Haiti, Antigua, and Saint Kitts and Nevis.

Suicide is a tragic way of dying. Some well-known people who have taken their own life include the artist Vincent van Gogh, the actor Robin Williams, the chef Anthony Bourdain, the writer Ernest Hemingway, the poet Sylvia Plath and the singer Kurt Cobain. The Golden Gate Bridge holds the un-lucky title of the number-one suicide landmark in the world. Since it opened in 1937, more than 1 300 people have jumped to their deaths from the bridge.

Men who commit suicide seem to use more violent meth-ods, like shooting or stabbing themselves or jumping to their death, while women tend to use more passive methods, like overdosing or gassing.

I find it very curious that in cases where people shoot themselves in the head, they hardly ever aim for their eyes, ears, or nose, and that people who jump from bridges or high buildings usually try to miss objects on the way down. It is almost as if they don't want to hurt themselves. Individuals who hang themselves often also tend to use padding between the rope and their neck. I have even seen prisoners – who don't have access to the Internet and couldn't have researched it – use padding. So, even when people know they are about to die, they try to avoid feeling physical pain.

Another curious fact about suicide cases is that during the autopsy we find that their stomachs are usually full. This indicates that they probably had a last meal before committing suicide.

The books *Final Exit* and *The Good Euthanasia Guide*, both by Derek Humphry, and *I'll See Myself Out, Thank You*, edited by Colin Brewer and Michael Irwin, have caused quite a lot of trouble for forensic pathologists, since they teach people how to kill themselves painlessly, quickly and efficiently.

Of the newest ways to commit suicide is with dry ice (the solid form of carbon dioxide). Typically, the person buys a chunk of dry ice, seals the bathroom door and falls asleep with the chunk of dry ice in his or her arms. Sometimes, there will be a warning on the door: 'Be careful when you enter this bathroom – carbon dioxide gas!'[41] I have also observed trends in suicide cases. For example, you may see gassing cases for months, where people gas themselves in their vehicles. Petrol seems to be more popular than diesel as a method of gassing, despite it being more expensive, as the higher octane of petrol ensures a quicker death than the lower octane of diesel. Then, for no apparent reason, we will see no gassings for months. But suddenly there will be an increase in the number of hangings. At times, I have seen so many hangings that I wanted to go to every hardware store and tell the manager that buying rope should be as stringently regulated as buying a handgun.

On one single wintry day, the autopsy cutting list had ten hangings from all over town. These people neither knew nor communicated with one another. Perhaps a suggestion went out 'into the ether', almost like the suicides of Robin Williams or Anthony Bourdain – and then, by means of the law of social proof, people committed suicide in sympathy with their icons.

In the four months after Robin Williams' suicide in August 2014, Centers for Disease Control data revealed that there were 18 690 suicides in the US – significantly more than the 16 849 suicides that past data and trends would have predicted for that particular period.

You do not have to be a medical doctor to help save someone's life. If someone is behaving very differently and their true self is not shining through, sit down with them and talk to them. Remember, you can always refer them to a professional. It helps to be mindful and to take an interest in those around you.

You should also be aware of someone's mood – especially if they regularly seem to be on an extreme high. A person's mood is like a sine wave. If their mood goes up to positive 95 per cent, you can be sure that it will drop to negative 95 per cent in eight to twelve hours' time. That is the theory of bipolar disorder: what goes up, must come down.

If you take a psychostimulant such as cocaine, you will

experience an euphoric high, but eight to twelve hours later your mood will crash and you will need another 'hit' to experience the same high. The same goes for caffeine – if you are addicted to caffeine, you need a kick in the morning (another 'hit').

The reason I am discussing this is because most people with crushing depression have been exposed to some or other form of psychostimulant in the past (amphetamines, cocaine, ecstasy tablets, even supra-pharmacological dosages of caffeine). Often, emergency medicine physicians, general practitioners and clinicians do not see people's downs, but we as forensic pathologists do, because they present with suicidal death.

I have had the misfortune of reading hundreds of suicide notes – about 20 per cent of all suicide victims are considerate enough to leave a note of sorts. Some of the notes I have read are extremely personal, emotional and very sad; they leave you with an intense feeling of hopelessness.

I have seen suicide notes written on mobile phones, computers and even on a wall, like graffiti. Often, they are handwritten. Some are verbal (where the person who committed suicide left a recorded message for someone). Others are sent via text message or voice note. Nowadays, we are also seeing a lot of suicide notes being posted on social media.

Over the years I have picked up a few common traits in the notes I have read. The note is usually addressed to someone in particular who is very dear to that person, and it is often written in emotional language. The notes almost always contain the words 'I' and 'you'. There is almost always a confession of sorts. For instance the person would write, 'I'm sorry for . . .', 'I can't go on like this . . .', 'I wish you well . . .' or 'Tell [this person] that . . .'

The note could contain end-of-life directives, for example, 'My banking details are . . .' or 'My PIN number is . . .' Mostly, the note contains a mobile phone number indicating who should be called when the body is discovered. At times, we have to actively search for the note – it may be crumpled up in the smallest pocket of the person's jeans, or even in their underwear or in a shoe or a sock.

The average suicide note is either *very* short or *very* long. When the note is handwritten, it is either extremely untidy or very neat. We are usually quite sceptical about typed suicide notes (as they could have been typed by someone else).

One day, I performed an autopsy on a teenage girl who had jumped from the eleventh storey of a building. Her suicide note was four pages long. In it, she explained that she had fallen pregnant, which was the reason she had killed herself. On another day, I performed an autopsy on a twenty-seven-year-old man who had hanged himself. He had underlying heart disease and was really sick. His suicide note was only three lines long.

When I consider all the different ways in which people die, it breaks my heart. I am always plagued by two questions: Could these deaths have been prevented? And, why am I seeing the same type of death more than once?

11

Fighting crime with science

Over the years, South African society has become more and more emotionally blunted to crime and death. When we first heard about house robberies and hijackings, we were shocked. After a while, these crimes became fairly common. People started responding to them by saying things like, 'Well, at least no one was hurt.'

The problem is that hijacking, robbery, murder and any other attacks on innocent civilians represent pathology in society. The 'at least' response is pathological – it is an unnatural response to an unnatural situation. In my opinion, almost all of our problems begin with the words 'at least'. It is not a natural response to a natural situation – it is an unnatural response to an unnatural situation.

The thing is, the baseline of what is considered normal is constantly shifting. In fact, some refer to it as shifting baseline syndrome, which means that, over time, knowledge is lost about the state of the natural world because people don't perceive changes that are actually taking place. It is a type of change to how a system is measured, usually against previous reference points (baselines), which themselves may represent significant changes from an even earlier state of the system.

What is normal today? For instance, what is a normal forensic pathology case load for a forensic pathologist? Was the suicide rate always this high? Was homicide always this violent? At times, the numbers of the dead and the severity of the pathology seen at autopsy makes me think that I am living in a *Mad Max* movie.

When people ask me, 'What is killing South Africans?', my answer is simple: 'South Africans are killing South Africans. We are a country at war with itself.' This brings me back to the reason I went into forensic pathology – I wanted to help real victims. This is my silent and steady driver. Every time I hear of a crime, it boils my blood and I feel compelled to work harder and smarter to catch and outwit the criminals. It isn't always easy in these times, with the rights of criminals seemingly far outweighing the rights of civilians, when the burden of proof is so heavy and rich criminals seem to be able to buy their freedom with expensive defence lawyers. By proving scientifically that right is right, I do my bit to ensure that justice prevails.

There is simply no greater feeling than that of helping to catch a bad guy. Studying and working in forensic pathology has made me feel like something of a vigilante crime fighter. It gives me immeasurable pleasure to see criminals in handcuffs, heads bowed, being taken to their cells after a guilty verdict.

I am not physically strong. All I have is my mind, which I use to help fight crime and bullying, and to defeat evil. In the words of Rudyard Kipling: 'They copied all they could follow, but they couldn't copy my mind, / and I left 'em sweating and stealing, a year and a half behind.'

I have dealt with my fair share of criminals over the past decade, and not all of them were dead. Mr X was the head of one of the most dangerous syndicates in the country. He had been on Southern Africa's most wanted list for several years before he was finally caught. The charges against him included, but were not limited to, house robbery, hijacking, murder, assault, assault with grievous bodily harm, rape and kidnapping, and he was even implicated in rhino horn trafficking.

He had apparently escaped from prison twice before, but when I met him he was awaiting trial in one of the most secure prison facilities in the country. (The policeman who eventually captured Mr X was given a car as a reward.)

Apparently, Mr X had left a single droplet of blood at one crime scene. A reference blood sample was required from him for DNA testing in order to prove his presence at that specific scene. I was asked to draw the blood. Blood was also to be taken from him to test for a host of sexually transmitted diseases, because he had also been implicated in several rape cases.

I thought my last living patient was the British man with the asthma attack who smoked fifty cigarettes a day. I was now to meet another living patient.

When I arrived at the prison, I was met by the head of security, who briefed me on just how dangerous Mr X was. He was being kept in isolation, away from all the other prisoners, and was under what the head of security called 'extreme lockdown'. I was told how to behave, and even how to communicate with Mr X.

To get to Mr X, I would have to walk past all the other dangerous inmates in that particular prison block. I was warned to keep my hands in my pockets and not to make eye contact.

I was also warned to stay well away from the cells in case one of the prisoners grabbed me from within a cell and injured me or tried to strangle me against the prison bars.

I must confess that, after hearing this brief and what the police had told me about Mr X, shivers went down my spine. According to the stories, Mr X was an ex-child soldier from a neighbouring African country who had killed countless people and apparently had no social conscience. He had moved to South Africa and become involved in criminal activities. Apparently he was extremely successful, and had built up a small criminal empire.

With hands in my pockets, I slowly walked the block where the most dangerous criminals were kept. The smells and sounds of that prison block I cannot describe in words. I was shocked by the conditions: it seemed so overcrowded. I had heard that inmates rotated their bunk beds for six- to eight-hour sleep shifts because there weren't enough beds for all of them.

After passing door after door after door of concrete and iron, in what seemed like a labyrinth of passages, I finally arrived at Mr X's cell. I was escorted by three bulky prison guards, the most muscular prison officials I have ever had the privilege to meet. I could feel my heart pounding.

But the man who sat before me was the most insignificant-looking individual I had ever seen. This 40 kg slip of a man was just sitting there in his chair, looking as helpless as a sickly elderly person. He neither greeted me nor made any attempt at eye contact. He just sat there, passively, staring at the floor. He was only twenty-seven years old, but he had already lived the lives of many men.

I simply drew the blood from his arm, thanked him and left the prison.

Meeting Mr X was one of the biggest non-events of my career. I was expecting a Hannibal Lecter type from *Silence of the Lambs*, but what I saw before me was a person you wouldn't even notice if you walked past him in the street. By the way the police had built him up in my mind, he had become some near-mythological figure. This reaffirmed a very basic life lesson: it's not what you look like, but what you've done in your life that counts.

Later that week, his blood tests returned from the laboratory. He had tested positive for a whole range of tenacious sexually transmitted diseases. His DNA also matched the DNA of the blood found on the crime scene.

Prison is terrifying place, even in the daytime. A female colleague once attended a death scene at a high-security prison. The wardens had moved all the prisoners from the death scene to the courtyard three storeys below.

My colleague peered down at the courtyard from the third storey to look at all the prisoners as they talked, played dice and did weights. When her head appeared over the balcony, they all stopped what they were doing and gazed up at her – like one being. My colleague said it was one of the most eerie experiences of her life. She said that she felt very vulnerable at that moment.

My medical colleague Rob, who once served as a prison doctor, regaled me with another tale. He was called to examine a prisoner with a very strange complaint. Apparently this prisoner could squirt blood from his eyes. Rob informed me that prisoners typically devise all sort of tricks and tactics to scare the wardens and get admitted into sick bay. This particular prisoner used a sharp object to injure the mucosa of his nasal cavity. He then blocked his nostrils with his index finger and thumb, for the dripping blood to collect in his nasal cavity. He would then blow his nose, forcing the blood out of the nasolacrimal ducts, which open on the inner corner of the eyes, close to the lacrimal caruncles. This caused blood to squirt from his eyes.

Of the most intriguing things I have ever witnessed in a prison was the so-called 26s gang death salute, something very few people have ever witnessed. This is a chilling, choreographed, dance, which is almost, but not entirely, like the haka, the Maori ceremonial dance or challenge. The haka is a fierce display of tribal pride, strength and unity. Actions include violent foot-stamping, tongue protrusions and rhythmic body slapping, accompanied by a loud chant.

I was asked to attend to a death of a male in a high-security prison who had apparently hanged himself from the bars in his cell. These days, prisons are designed to be suicide proof. There are no longer bars in front of the windows, but mesh grilles. The toilets in prisons do not have chains or flushing handles as you would probably know them; instead, they have push buttons. Sometimes there are no toilets at all, just a pit in the floor. Even the beds have no places to tie a noose and are typically made of concrete.

Still, prisoners find ingenious methods of hanging themselves. I have seen prisoners hang themselves with shoelaces, clothing, and even toilet paper . . . If you weave toilet paper tightly enough, you can make an excellent noose ligature with which to hang yourself or strangle another person – after which you can simply flush it down the toilet.

Even the lights in the cells are designed in such a way that no noose can be tied to them – they are typically recessed. The showers' handles and nozzles are also designed to make it near impossible for someone to tie a noose to them. Despite this, I've seen a noose tied to a shower nozzle that extended from the wall at an acute downward angle. The prisoner had ingenuously turned the shower nozzle upwards, creating a 'hook' – onto which he tied the noose.

The prisoner whose death scene I had to attend was a 26s gang 'general'. He had hanged himself in his cell. After removing the body and the noose from the mesh grille, we had to get it from the upper floor of the prison to our mortuary vehicle, which was parked outside, three floors down. To get there, we had to carry the body across the courtyard. We covered the body with a blanket and put it on a body tray.

What I saw in the twenty or thirty minutes that followed was one of the most chilling and haunting experiences of my life. All the prisoners performed the same dance with military precision in their respective cells, even though they had not had the chance to practise or choreograph it. Every time the body of the deceased prisoner passed a cell, the inmates performed this death salute.

This 'dance' was so impressive and invoked such fear in me that I thought the Springbok rugby team should consider using it. That would surely give the All Blacks a run for their money.

I am particularly proud of a case in which my discovery and description of protective amulets not only helped the police to investigate an armed robbery, but also played a role in exposing an international terrorism syndicate. Once again, science and keen observations ruled the day.

But first, a word or two on protective amulets. From a lucky rabbit's foot to good luck charms or religious symbols like crosses or the icons of saints, people use various items to bring them good luck or to protect them from evil.[42]

In South Africa, the use of muti or protective amulets provided by traditional healers, or sangomas, is widespread. There is ancestor worship and a belief in the Tokoloshe, a mischievous evil spirit. It is therefore not surprising that I have found a vast number of good luck charms, protective amulets and body guards on bodies over the years. Apparently, the victims of the Marikana Massacre all wore good luck charms on their bodies and had scarification marks on their bodies from traditional healers, which were intended to make them bulletproof.

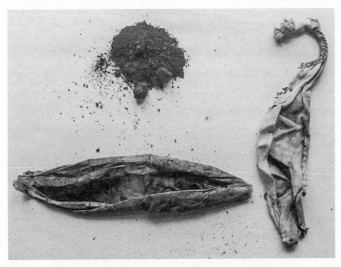

Over the years I have seen countless traditional strings, crucifixes and evil eyes, among other things, around the abdomens and wrists of the deceased.

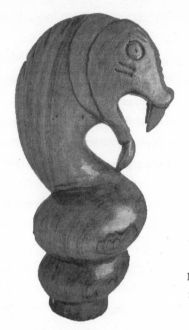

Nyami Nyami, the Zambezi
river god or Zambezi snake
spirit from Zimbabwe.

I do not understand all the traditional belief systems surrounding protective amulets and it is not my place to try to understand the intricacies surrounding them, but I do know that both innocent citizens and criminals use muti and amulets to protect or to heal themselves. The psychological impact that such amulets may have on the minds and actions of individuals needs to be studied further, but it is safe to assume that certain amulets could possibly make criminals more brazen.

In forensic practice all over the world, people are often found with some kind of lucky charm on their bodies. These lucky charms may take varied forms from country to country and culture to culture, but they are always endowed with helpful, magical properties. Sometimes, the charm is meant to protect its owner from bad luck; in other instances, it is intended to bring them good luck.

For millions of people all over the world, carrying a lucky charm or protective amulet brings a sense of calm and makes them less fearful. From the evil eye in Turkey to the beckoning cat in Japan, amulets have become good luck symbols for entire nations. And in remote parts of Africa, women often carry fertility figures in their clothing to increase their chances of becoming pregnant.

Often the contents of good luck charms may contain many strange and unusual substances. It may perhaps be unkind to say it, but if one were to do a retrospective study of all the

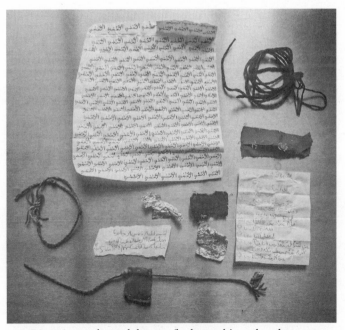

Protective amulets and charms – 'body guards' – such as these are believed to ward off bad luck or attract good fortune. *Photo: R Blumenthal*

good luck charms and amulets I have seen at the mortuary, it would appear that none of them worked in protecting their owners from unnatural death.

In my particular case, a group of six criminals were found at autopsy to be wearing good luck charms which, when opened, had Arabic writing on them. I had opened the amulets out of curiosity and found the writing on pieces of parchment-like paper.

What I had discovered was a type of *taweez*. A *taweez* is a locket or good luck charm that contains certain prayers or scriptures. This led the police to investigate deeper; the amulets were found to connect the six criminals to a well-known international terrorism syndicate.

Apparently, the six men were funding the syndicate through cash-in-transit robberies in South Africa. It was through my curiosity about their amulets that the link to the syndicate was made.

12

The perfect murder . . .

Another question I am frequently asked is, 'What is the perfect murder?' Over the years I have consulted the most brilliant minds on this matter. It amazes me how seriously people have thought about it. Their answers often astound me!

I have heard some truly far-fetched suggestions – from shooting people with ice bullets to using strange types of poisoning agents. The bottom line is that many of these methods will leave some or other trace of evidence.

People have also shared a few far-fetched ideas about how to dispose of a body. This has included dissolving bodies in strong acid, and disposing of them at pig farms. It would certainly be impossible to perform an autopsy with no body, and would complicate things for us forensic pathologists.

To my mind, the perfect murder could take place in a scenario in which one of the partners in a relationship or marriage starts to make excessive demands on the other, be they financial, psychological, emotional or physical. If that person has an underlying comorbid disease, such as high blood pressure, diabetes, a tendency to arrhythmias, etc., they could eventually die from a coronary thrombosis, arrhythmia, or myocardial ischaemia. If you were unaware of the background, you would most likely certify the death as due to natural causes, when in reality it was a result of unnatural causes.[43]

When considering the perfect murder, you always need to be on the lookout for what is most common. As I often tell my students, an uncommon presentation of a common thing is still more common than an uncommon thing. If you are a bird-watcher, for example, a common bird with unusual feathers is still more common than a bird from overseas that has been swept off course. Therefore, before you consider a weird, unusual, crazy solution, consider an abnormal presentation of a common solution.

There are two basic rules in the field of forensics: assume that the murderers are cleverer than you, and assume that they know all the methods. They may have downloaded the latest forensic journals, or could even own copies of all the forensic homicide investigation books. They could also have watched the television show *CSI* or *The Mentalist*. Never assume that they are stupid.

Before considering a crazy type of murder, consider a run-of-the-mill murder. But even before you do this, consider murder – *always* consider murder. Even when it seems like a natural, accidental or suicidal death, always keep in mind the possibility of murder.

What would intimidate you more: being told to solve a problem, or being told find out if there is a problem? Solving problems could be described as easy compared to figuring out whether there is a problem in the first place. As a forensic pathologist, you obviously never want to miss a murder. This is probably the gravest mistake we can make in our field. Therefore, we treat every single case as a possible murder.

Certain homicides are known as simulacrum of the norm murders – in other words, murders that are made to look like a suicide, an accident or a natural death. Detecting these presents the greatest challenge. I like to use an example from the world of sleight-of-hand card magic to explain this. Cards are usually dealt off the top of a pack, but card sharks can 'second deal' – deal the card second from the top of a pack, pretending that it is the top card. Unless you have seen thousands of normal deals, as well as thousands of second deals, you would likely not notice second dealing. The subtleties of the grip, the speed of dealing and the technique of dealing the second card could give away the card shark's second deal.

The perfect second deal would be akin to the perfect murder. The second deal would either have to be *really* good, or it would have to be presented to a layperson, who would assume it was a normal deal off the top of the pack.

For instance, you get typical and atypical hanging cases. Is this a real suicide, or actually a crafty murder? Even if you have never seen a hanging before in your life, if you were to hang yourself, you would do it in a typical way. Forensic pathologists look for these typical findings. If you were to kill someone and then hang him or her up, it would look slightly different – it would be an atypical hanging.

Criminals are always on the lookout for newer, more sophisticated and craftier ways to dispatch their victims. Obviously, the most difficult cases are the ones in which there is no body to examine. The legal aspects surrounding such cases are complex. However, these murders are by no means perfect. Murderers have been caught and convicted, despite the fact that there is no body to autopsy.

There may be no dead body, but there may be a body of evidence: 'corpus delicti' is 'body of the crime' in Latin. In its original sense, the body in question refers not to a corpse but to the body of essential facts that, taken together, prove that a crime has been committed.

As a forensic pathologist, you need to keep abreast of technological advances. Homicide by mobile phone is one example. A case has been reported in which someone hacked a medical device via mobile phone. In this instance, the medical device was an insulin pump, hacked to deliver a supra-pharmacological dose of insulin to the patient, who died. Nowadays, technology companies have to ensure that medical devices are hack-proof.[44]

Then there are new kinds of drone that are very small, and can be programmed to recognise someone's facial features. Engineers have created what is known as swarm technology. These small drones could be armed with a small amount of explosive material, for example, and could kill whole populations without inflicting any damage to infrastructure or buildings.

Of course, new technologies can also work in forensic pathologists' favour and help us to catch criminals. So-called laboratories-on-a-chip are an example. If you find a droplet of blood on a death scene, you can place it in a hand-held device, which will phenotype the blood and state whether the owner of that blood has blonde hair or blue eyes. This can help investigators to identify the murderer's physical attributes at the death scene.

Experts are now working on removing fingerprints from a person's neck in strangulation cases, and also on the timing of the fingerprint. They hope to establish the time at which the suspect touched the victim. Some experts are even working on determining the suspect's diet from their fingerprint.[45]

There is also new facial recognition software, and software that analyses a person's gait, with which scientists can now identify a person from the way they walk.[46]

Scientists have even found new and innovative ways of retrieving all the data from a mobile phone that has been in a house fire. Imagine a mobile phone spending six hours, at table-height, in a house fire, burning at 450–650 °C. Scientists may still be able to extract data from the charred device.[47]

Some scientists are even looking at the weaponisation of lightning. Yes: imagine being purposefully struck by lightning. Experts are working on lasers that create ionic channels between cloud and ground, through which a lightning bolt may strike.

But generally speaking, not that much is new in murder. People still mostly die from firearms, blunt force trauma and sharp force trauma. The biblical ways of killing and dying are still very much alive and well in these modern times.

In martial art or hand-to-hand combat classes, the teacher (sensei) will often say, 'Come at me like this,' or 'Come at me like that.' The student will then try to attack the teacher – and most often end up flat on their face, or in some or other kind of hold. The reality is that real assaults are not 'sensei compliant'. The attackers rarely come at you like this, or like that. The assaults we see on a day-to-day basis are so quick and so extremely violent that the poor victim never stood a chance. Most of the murders we see involve the element of surprise.

Something I have noticed is that poisoning as a method of

murder seems to be working its way out of society, because of sophisticated new developments in poison detection methods. Machines like gas chromatography–mass spectrometry and liquid chromatography–mass spectrometry are the gold standards for forensic substance identification, because they positively identify the presence of a particular substance. These machines are so specific that they can even detect trace amounts of pesticides used against flies in the mortuary, which may have accidentally settled on the dead body despite having been sprayed from many metres away.

Apart from the question about the perfect murder, people often also ask me how I manage to endure the smell at an autopsy. Let me start off by saying that the smell at autopsy is by no means worse than some of the other smells in medicine.

I recently received an e-mail from an old veterinary surgeon, in which he described his life in retirement. He explained how he had pondered the difference between the smell of a rotting cow and a rinkhals (a South African snake) that he had killed when it had tried to slip in through his kitchen door. The smell of the cow, he wrote, was 'reasonably acceptable', but the smell of the snake was 'unbearable'. He wrote, 'The decomposing carcasses of carnivorous animals seem to stink far worse than those of herbivores. If that is the case, do humans whose eating habits are vegan smell differently after leaving this beautiful planet?'

There is a whole literature on the topic of smell at autopsy. As I have explained, there are many different – unpleasant – odours after death, and they are caused by a multitude of different factors. Post-mortem odour is typically caused by different amines, such as putrescine and cadaverine – foul-smelling, organic chemicals caused by the breakdown of amino acids. These two compounds are largely responsible for the foul odour of putrefying flesh.

Forensic scientists are currently trying to use the different amines to determine time since death. Depending on the stage of decay (early decay, green decay, black decay, or the stage of butyric fermentation), different odours may be experienced from the same corpse.

Certain anaerobic bacteria produce hydrogen sulphide post-mortem, which is quite offensive indeed. Hydrogen sulphide gas may even cause death if inhaled in significant amounts. Other bacteria produce methane gas, which is flammable post-mortem.

The question of whether carnivores, herbivores and omni-vores smell different after death may have a subtle bearing on this topic. That herbivore dung may be less offensive than car-nivore dung has less to do with evolutionary biology than with the fact that carnivores ingest blood. Melaena stools in humans (from an upper gastrointestinal tract bleed caused by swal-lowed blood travelling down the intestines) have a particu-larly offensive odour. Herbivores do not wish to be detected by carnivores, so their dung may be less offensive.

Carnivores also tend to be 'dirtier' than herbivores. Lions, for example, are filthy creatures. As mentioned earlier, I have performed autopsies on deaths due to lion scratches. Always wear gloves when you handle lion dung.

So, what are the worst odours I have ever experienced? Going from bad to worse, in fifth position would be a living patient with melaena stools. Melaena refers to thick, black, tarry stools that usually occur as a result of upper gastro-intestinal bleeding. The stools are often difficult to flush away, due to the alteration and degradation of blood by intestinal enzymes and have a very specific odour. You can smell them from down the hallway.

Coming in at number four would be a living burns patient, lying in a burns unit hospital bed, with secondary *Pseudomonas aeruginosa* infection. This Gram-negative infection has a classic bittersweet, grape-like smell, which is slightly astringent.

The third-worst smell is a dead body in the black stage of fermentation, or perhaps a dead body in the stage of butyric fermentation. This is a body that has been decomposing for about a month. It has a classic gorgonzola cheese-like smell.

The second-worst smell is a living female patient with cervical cancer.

And the absolutely worst smell in medicine, in my opinion, is that of a perianal abscess. I have experienced one or two of these abscesses in my career. The smell attaches itself to your hair and clothes for about a week.

Imagine incising into a perianal abscess. Warm, custard-like pus bursts forth and then oozes outwards. With it, a positive pressure wave of odour sends you reeling backwards like the main character in *The Matrix*. Imagine a skunk on steroids – it gets your eyes watering, and sends your lungs into pre-bronchospasm. Nothing – I repeat, nothing – comes close to the stench of a perianal abscess.

However, I must admit that, when all is said and done, the field of odourology or smellology remains highly subjective. There are certain things in my line of work that you simply have to deal with; bad odour is one of them.

Here's a handy tip, though: a cup of granulated chlorine placed in a mortuary fridge destroys most bad odours. Granulated chlorine works better than any air freshener. I don't know whether it's a myth, but apparently a cup of granulated chlorine placed in a roof also deters roof rats.

To think that some humans are born with anosmia, or loss of smell. They can't even appreciate the good smells.

Nothing seems to fascinate people more than stomach contents at autopsy. You only have to listen to a few high-profile court cases to understand the public's morbid fascination with stomach contents.

Forensic pathologists have the unenviable task of meticulously having to go through the entire stomach contents of the dead. One day, I did an autopsy on a motor vehicle accident driver and found the victim's blue, semi-chewed gum among the stomach contents. Clearly, he had swallowed the gum at the time of the accident.

From personal experience, the most common food rests I have seen in the stomachs of South Africans are farinaceous food rests – in other words, those made of flour or meal. One of the strangest cases on which an older colleague of mine worked involved a railway track victim. The grossly mutilated body was found on the tracks; only slips of skin and crushed bone remained. The victim was unrecognisable.

When my colleague opened what was left of the stomach, he found a crumpled-up piece of paper with a note that said: 'My name is X, the following people are coming to kill me: X.' The deceased had written his murderers' names on a piece of paper and swallowed it before he was killed. He managed to put his murderers away from beyond the grave.

Often, you will find semi-digested pill rests in the stomachs of those who have overdosed on mixed medication. As mentioned earlier, you may also find Temik (aldicarb), which looks like multiple, small, crushed, grey-black granules, admixed in the gastric contents. Sometimes, the stomach contents may have a chemical smell, which betrays the diagnosis.

Then you get the really crazy stuff: bezoars. When a tightly packed mass of undigested or partially digested material builds up in the digestive tract, it is known as a bezoar, and it can cause a blockage. Bezoars occur in animals and humans of all age groups, and are most commonly found in the stomach. The following bezoars may be found:

- Phytobezoars are the most common type. They are composed of indigestible vegetable fibres.
- Diospyrobezoars are a type of phytobezoar composed of persimmon fruit.
- Trichobezoars are composed of hair and food particles, and can end up weighing several kilograms.
- Pharmacobezoars are composed of medications that have not dissolved.
- Lactobezoars are composed of milk protein and mucus.
- Foreign-body bezoars contain material such as tissue paper, plastic, polystyrene foam cups and parasitic worms.

One of the strangest swallowing deaths I have ever encountered involved a psychiatric patient who had been storing 40 cm × 20 cm newspaper clippings under his bed. They were on topics that did not seem related to anything. One told of the Kruger National Park fires, for example, while another described some or other weather phenomenon.

Be that as it may, one day this psychiatric patient decided to swallow all of the newspaper articles he had saved in one swift go. When I performed the autopsy, I found a papier-mâché impression of his entire upper swallowing tract, and his stomach was full of newspaper. Death was probably due to a mixture of INCA, asphyxiation, and/or pica, which we return to later.

Rabies, a contagious and fatal viral disease of dogs and other mammals, sometimes causes the infected animal to eat strange things. My veterinary pathology colleagues have told me how they have found rocks and stones in the stomachs of rabies-infected dogs.

Once, we were presented with the case of an adult male who died suddenly and unexpectedly. Upon X-raying his body, multiple screws were noted in the left breast pocket. However, upon external examination no screws were found in his left pocket. Clearly, the screws were in his stomach. One of the screws had penetrated the stomach wall and had caused his death.

Pica is an eating disorder typically defined as the persistent ingestion of non-nutritive substances for at least one month, at an age for which this behaviour is developmentally inappropriate. It can be benign, or it can have life-threatening consequences. In this particular situation, the consequences were fatal.

One of the assistants who had helped to dissect the body turned around and gave me a naughty look. 'Seems like he enjoyed the odd screw!' he said, with a mischievous grin.

In this field, you have to maintain a sense of humour, despite the many dark things you see.

Screws are not the only strange objects that have been found in unexpected places in the human body, however. The following story was relayed to me by a clinical colleague Nicholas. Once, when he was on duty in emergency medicine, a man came in for an examination. According to my colleague, the guy looked a little sheepish.

In the centre of his forehead was a colourful Mickey Mouse plaster.

'What happened?' my colleague asked.

'Last of last night . . .' the patient said, with a triple hop of his right index finger. 'Last of last night, I felt something hit me in my head. So I put a plaster on it.'

My colleague proceeded to remove the Mickey Mouse plaster. Pus exuded from the wound. X-ray examination showed a 9 mm projectile lodged within the man's frontal sinus. His brain was completely uninjured. He had sustained a gunshot entrance wound to his forehead – and thought it fitting to cover it with a Mickey Mouse plaster.

The rest of the story revealed itself the following day when police officers came to the hospital looking for a suspected car hijacker.

'Last of last night,' began the one policeman, with exactly the same triple hop of his right index finger. 'Last of last night, there was a hijacking, and we could have sworn we shot one suspect, but he disappeared.'

The fact that the policeman and the hijacker had used the same unusual opening line and the same right index finger triple hop was beyond belief. But even more startling was the fact that the hijacker had covered a 9 mm gunshot entrance wound successfully with a Mickey Mouse plaster.

13

Animals and death

Pets and other animals have a lot to teach us, if we watch them carefully enough. When you arrive at a death scene, you always look at what the pets are up to. For example, if a dog cowers, with its tail tucked tightly between its legs, beware of the owner. It could be a sign that the owner is an abusive person.

I have a number of stories that relate to pets and animals at death scenes. The first is of a woman who had been murdered by her lodger. I will not go into the grizzly details of the forensic examination, but she had been stabbed multiple times.

When we arrived at the scene, the deceased's four dachshunds were standing over her body, defending it viciously and destroying a lot of the evidence. There were bloody paw prints everywhere. Every time we tried to come close to the body, the dogs attacked us.

The one policeman offered to run to the shops and buy something to lure the dogs away from the body. He returned with a Russian sausage; it goes without saying that this tactic did not work.

Eventually we phoned the police's dog unit, which dispatched a dog whisperer to the scene.

Shortly afterwards, a female captain arrived at the scene. Somehow, she managed to find out the names of the dogs. Three minutes later, she walked away from the death scene with the alpha dog tightly wrapped in a blanket over her shoulder and the other three dogs in tow. It was a goosebumps moment, something you don't get to see every day.

In another case, I arrived at the scene of death of a man who had been found dead in his bedroom. His throat had apparently been slit. Outside, beyond the police tape, I passed his elderly neighbours, who were holding and petting his two lapdogs.

I examined the scene and the deceased, and immediately realised what I was dealing with. There was indeed a large open wound on the anterior aspect of the neck. Damage caused by canine and rodent predators is usually obvious. There is local removal of a large amount of flesh, and usually evidence of teeth marks. Rats and cats leave a crenated edge, the post-mortem nature of which is obvious from the lack of bleeding.

The man had died from a heart attack, but the injuries to the anterior aspect of his neck were caused by his two dogs that had been in the room with him when he had died. It is a sad fact that pets often feed on their owners after death. I could not bring myself to mention this to the kind-looking, elderly neighbours who were petting his dogs.

In another incident, a light aircraft crashed in the mountains. The pilot and co-pilot – apparently the only two people in the plane – were both charred beyond recognition. Both bodies were carefully removed and autopsies performed on the remains.

The following day, we got a phone call from someone who was on the scene. They had found another burned skull under the wreckage, but no accompanying body. We asked the police to bring it to us for examination. When we examined it, we established that it was actually that of a dassie (rock hyrax). Interestingly, the burned remains of a dassie look very similar to those of a burned human skull.

On another occasion, I arrived at a death scene where a woman had allegedly fallen down a flight of stairs. The moment I got there, a boerboel ran up to me and urinated on my leg. To me, this was abnormal animal behaviour.

The husband of the deceased wife was only too helpful on the scene. He pointed out the wife's body at the bottom of the flight of stairs. When I performed the autopsy, I found bruises on the inner aspects of her thighs and perineum – injuries that would be hard to induce by falling down a flight of stairs. When people fall down stairs, their injuries are more likely to be found on the outer aspects of the body.

When the police investigated the case, it turned out that the husband had murdered his wife and tried to make it look like an accident. The dog's behaviour initially alerted me to possible pathology on the scene – something wasn't right. In retrospect, I realised that the dog was the real hero in this case.

One morning, a fifty-seven-year-old man from a small town on the banks of the Vaal River heard his dog barking outside. He opened the front door to see what was going on. The next moment, a yellow mongoose jumped up at him and bit him on his wrist. It would not let go. The man then strangled the mongoose to death while it was latched to his wrist.

An emergency doctor flushed his wound, gave him a tetanus injection and put him on antibiotics. The man took the dead mongoose to the local veterinary institute, where the veterinary pathologist diagnosed rabies.

In South Africa, human rabies is due to infection with the classic rabies virus. The yellow mongoose is the commonest vector, except in KwaZulu-Natal, the Eastern Cape, Mpumalanga and Limpopo where dogs are responsible for most bites. Rabies is always fatal in humans but can be prevented by timeous administration of post-exposure prophylaxis.

The man was therefore immediately admitted to hospital and treated for possible rabies infection. He started having pain in the arm, fever and headache, followed by an illness characterised by periods of lucidity, hallucinations and confusion. He died three weeks later, despite receiving full post-exposure prophylaxis. The clinicians were of the opinion that the mongoose had bitten directly into a nerve, or that the man had been infected by a particularly virulent strain of rabies.

Due to the law of the land, this kind of death is considered an unnatural death in South Africa. Arrangements were made for a medicolegal post-mortem examination. Due to the highly infectious nature of this kind of case, it was arranged to perform the autopsy under extreme biosafety conditions. This entailed the autopsy being performed on superabsorbent sponge. The head of the deceased had to be covered in a plastic bag and no oscillating head saw was to be used, as it could have caused bone dust to be aerosolised. Instead, a manual hacksaw was used to open the head. Such highly infectious cases demand that no aerosol-generating procedures are used.

As mentioned earlier, certain viruses may be recovered for up to two weeks from the human corpse. The autopsy on a rabies case is considered very high risk.

Half of the brain was double bagged and put on ice before it was sent in a police van to the National Institute of Communicable Diseases (NICD). The other half of the brain was placed in formalin for forensic histology examination.

Later that afternoon, the NICD phoned to tell me that this was one of the highest viral loads of rabies that they had seen in a long time. Upon microscopic examination of the brain, multiple Negri bodies were identified within the neurons. Negri bodies are the pathognomonic findings which prove that this was an *ipso facto* rabies case. My two colleagues and I were strongly advised to go for full post-exposure treatment.

Animal rabies is endemic in South Africa and causes about ten to thirty laboratory-confirmed human deaths annually. It is likely that the number of actual human cases is significantly higher, with patients either dying in the community or the disease going unrecognised by health professionals and regarded as a possible case of any encephalitis-type illness.

I have seen several strange rabies cases over the years. One gentleman in the Drakensberg was apparently petting a rabbit when it apparently nibbled on his skin. A month later, he died of rabies. Another strange rabies incident happened in the small town of Muldersdrift, a popular destination for weddings outside Johannesburg. Apparently, a rabid jackal walked into a church at one of the wedding venues and licked one of the congregants. Fortunately, the congregant did not contract rabies.

Africa is full of scavengers that help to clean up the bush. There are hyenas, rats, mice, genets, jackals, fish, crabs, vultures, scavenging birds, and lots of stray dogs.

Often, a body is found in the middle of the veld with the ears, nose, fingers, toes or external genitalia missing. The first thought that passes through the mind of an investigator is that this could be a muti murder, since these appendages may have been used to produce traditional medicine.

The key to identifying a post-mortem predator injury is the lack of vital reaction, which means that the wounds do not look like they occurred during life: the wounds do not bleed, there is no swelling and there are no signs of healing.

One particular tale comes to mind, which I have not yet managed to fully verify. The story was told to me by a forensic colleague who practises way up in the northern part of the country, close to the Kruger National Park. The head of an adult female was discovered with no body and no nose, lying alone in the middle of the bush.

The surrounding area had been searched – there were no signs of the rest of her body. The case was quite a mystery – it almost looked as if her head had been dropped from the sky. Even the police dogs who were sent to scour the area could not find any further remains.

'What was the cause of death?' the ranger, who had discovered the head during his normal duties, asked my colleague.

My colleague was at a loss for words. The cause of death was impossible to establish; it was determined to be 'unascertainable at autopsy examination alone'. The diagnosis was obfuscated by the severe post-mortem predation. Initial impressions, on the face of it, seemed to suggest that wild animals had eaten, digested, scavenged, and scattered the rest of her body. The woman could have been a refugee who was trying to cross through the Kruger from Mozambique to South Africa. Perhaps she had been attacked by wild animals.

'What was the cause of death?' the ranger asked my colleague again.

He looked the ranger in the eye, took a deep breath and said slowly, 'Nobody knows!' (No body, no nose.)

This story brings me to a key point. Forensic pathologists are not miracle workers. While we always try our best, unfortunately we cannot solve every case. In about 10 to 15 per cent of all forensic autopsies one finds nothing macroscopically, and nothing on microscopy or toxicology. There are many cases where the diagnosis remains GOK – God only knows.

For example, a person could die from an electrolyte, metabolic or endocrine abnormality. In these scenarios, there could be absolutely nothing to find with the naked eye. All the organs in the body will seem normal.

Junior pathologists, wanting to impress senior pathologists, will try to push for an ethereal diagnosis. They may even find things that are not really there. They may, then, have a no-diagnosis rate of about 5 per cent. Older pathologists learn to doubt more as they get older, and could therefore have a no-diagnosis rate of about 20 per cent.

Unlike in clinical medicine, forensic cases cannot be triaged. In other words, in clinical medicine cases are assigned according to the degree of urgency of wounds or illnesses. This decides the order of treatment of a large number of patients and/or casualties. But in forensic pathology, the simplest cases may turn out to be the most complex – and the most complex may turn out to be the simplest. This is why, in forensics, you don't give supposedly easy cases to the juniors and supposedly complex cases to the seniors. It simply does not work like that.

For example, you could be presented with a pedestrian vehicle accident case but it could turn out to be a complex rape and homicide. Or, police may discover the body of a dead female dumped on the side of the road. Initially you could suspect a complex rape and homicide, but in fact it is an unwitnessed pedestrian vehicle accident.

There are other scenarios in which autopsy findings prove negative – for example, when a person dies due to positional asphyxia. Imagine they had tried entering a building through, say, a window and got stuck on the window ledge at the level of their stomach. In another scenario, someone could have fallen over and got their head trapped in a corner of a bed or cupboard. If the person was drunk at the time, or sedated, their breathing may have been compromised, leading to death.

In such instances, the scene of death is critically important. You need to see the body in the exact position at the time of death – *in situ*, so to speak – or diagnosis becomes virtually impossible. No matter how advanced the mortuary equipment, or how experienced the pathologist, it won't be possible to diagnose positional asphyxia in a mortuary.

Forensics is about being in the right state of mind on a daily basis to solve puzzles. You could say that we are in the business of puzzle solving.

Consider sudden infant death syndrome (SIDS), which is defined as 'the sudden death of an infant less than 1 year of age that remains unexplained after a complete autopsy and death scene investigation, and remains the most common cause of death in the post-perinatal period in countries with a relatively low infant mortality rate'.[48]

Most SIDS deaths take place between the ages of one month and six months, with a peak at two months. There is a slight preponderance in males. SIDS tends to be more common in the colder and the wetter months. The essence of SIDS is that the deaths are unexpected, and autopsy reveals no adequate cause.

Over the past decades, forensic pathologists have tested for everything they can possibly think of as a cause of SIDS – from house mites, botulism, prolonged sleep apnoea and spinal haemorrhages to various metabolic defects, hyperthermia and viral bronchiolitis. SIDS remains one of the greatest puzzles in modern forensic medicine. Perhaps SIDS is caused by something we cannot see because we don't know what to look for. Or perhaps we cannot see it because it is simply not visible.[49]

The question then becomes, how much time and money should be spent on a case before you give up? In approximately 15 per cent of infants who present clinically as SIDS deaths, an adequate cause of death may ultimately be demonstrated with thorough investigation. However, the remaining 85 per cent of cases will remain obscure and be confirmed as SIDS.

I once had to do an autopsy on a body that had gone through a wood chipper. Needless to say, this kind of case can be very difficult and time-consuming to investigate. It required absolute dedication to comb meticulously through the human remains to try to solve the puzzle.

Having to settle down and solve puzzles is what forensic

pathology is all about. At times, the puzzle seems unsolvable. It is almost as if it has a million pieces. In that moment, you might feel overwhelmed by an intense melancholy, almost as if you are staring into an abyss.

But then you simply remind yourself: every puzzle starts with one single piece.

14

Life in the witness box

I have spent countless hours in the witness box, testifying in front of judges and magistrates. I have been examined and cross-examined. At times, I have felt like I was on trial myself; take the following example of a line of questioning to which I was once subjected.

'You say the brain *appeared* pale?' the prosecutor in the case asked me in a provocative tone. 'What do you mean *appeared* pale, Doctor? Am I pale? Are you pale? Is the stenographer pale? Is your shirt pale? What exactly do you mean by *appeared* pale, Doctor?'

The prosecutor was relentless. As I've often said, there is no such thing as a perfect murder. There is, however, such a thing as a perfect lawyer.

You have to remain very composed in the witness box. You need to stand up, speak up, and – when necessary – shut up. No personal opinions may be given – only hard, scientific, factual evidence. The courts are overwhelmed; it is not uncommon to review a 2007 case in 2019.

I have spent many hours driving to small courtrooms in small rural towns, only to arrive to the case having been cancelled at the last minute. I have heard a multitude of reasons:

the lawyer is not present, the lawyer has back spasm. The stenographer is not present. The witness is not present. And the most frequent reason: a translator is not present (the South African Constitution recognises eleven official languages).

It is not uncommon for the accused to change their name in the holding cell, and for the wrong person to be standing in the dock. Criminals use every trick in the book to delay court proceedings. Dockets have been known to go missing, creating delays in court proceedings.

It is obviously very frustrating when cases are postponed. An entire day may be wasted, but being a servant of the courts, this unfortunately comes with the territory. I merely have to smile and go back to the mortuary.

The nature of litigation seems to be one of hurry up and wait. Legal actions sometimes have a tendency to resolve with or without the help of the forensic expert. Sometimes you are well prepared for a gruelling cross-examination and the matter is suddenly resolved prior to, or immediately after, the trial having commenced. At other times, you may end up giving testimony for hours about something you deemed trivial, and for which you were therefore not prepared.

I find that a lot of time is wasted going to courts when a written medicolegal opinion would have sufficed. Some days, I wonder whether the theatre of court proceedings is not merely a type of therapy for aggrieved families. I have also noticed that there seem to be people who are professional court attendees and who attend court on a daily basis, seeing it as some kind of reality television. They do not seem to have jobs; I get the sense that they do it for fun.

Once, I got called to court because an accused, who was

defending himself, wanted me to read the entire autopsy report to him in front of the court and explain every detail through a translator. As you can imagine, this took a significant amount of time. After I had read my report and explained it to him in plain language, the judge asked the accused whether he had any questions or comments, to which he replied, 'No.'

Most of the lawyers I know are smokers. I do not blame them. The day-to-day grind of the local criminal justice system can be extremely stressful.

I have been involved in a number of serious medicolegal cases. One day, I was in the witness box being thoroughly interrogated about an electrocution case. A young boy had gone in for a tonsillectomy and woken up with third-degree burns on the aspects of the skin just below and behind both knees. The assumption was that the wounds had probably been caused by electrical contact with the metal operating table while undergoing diathermy (electrical surgical cauterisation).

The following questions were posed to me in the witness box:

- Would the diathermy in the present case have been mono- or bipolar?
- What would inadequate preparation or positioning of the patient entail?
- What risks or harm would diathermy create?
- What is arcing injury?
- Would a surge in current cause a burn injury?
- Does difference in the size of the patient make a difference as to the extent of the burn (or whether a burn will, in fact, occur)?

- Why would a poorly insulated neutral electrode result in a burn?

The questions were incredibly well researched and I could not help but be impressed with the lawyers. It is beyond the scope of this book to go into the specifics of this case; it is enough to say that it entailed hours and hours of high-level interrogation.

At the end of the day, you do the best you can. You should never take court proceedings personally, even if you do not like the outcome of the trial personally. You are not there to 'win' the case. Your duty as a forensic pathologist is to help the judge understand the science that is relevant to the case.

On the stand, courtesy and good manners will stand you in good stead. Your body language has an impact, which means that you should stand up straight and dress appropriately. You should answer questions directly and succinctly, and be attentive and confident. You should also try to educate all who are present. You may need to refresh your memory before you testify, so you need to take a look at your original notes. Be honest and simply state the facts.

It is also very important not to put on an act. Posturing is seriously frowned upon. Never underestimate your audience, and never dramatise. And most importantly, do not wear out your welcome.[50]

In my job, I deal with some of the worst types of criminals and the worst kinds of evil. These are the ones who murder, who rape and who steal. I have seen some truly horrific crimes over the years. Just off the top of my head, I have seen women and children ironed with a hot iron by their attackers before they were killed. This was during a house robbery.

I have seen hijackers humiliate their victims for fun, before dispatching them. One hijacker locked his victim in the boot of a car and never released him. The victim died from neglect, thirst and possibly starvation. We also often see victims who have been thrown into the boot, and the car then set alight.

I have even performed autopsies on people who have been beheaded. In some cases, beheading was the cause of death; in others, the body was beheaded after death.

As I have said before, my sole mission in life is to try to take these villains down. But it is not always easy. Large sums of money will cause the brightest and richest to seek out the smallest of loopholes in cases.

Once, I was intensely cross-examined by a defence lawyer about a deceased woman's eyebrows. They were tattooed eyebrows, a fact that I had missed at autopsy. In my own defence, the eyebrows were so expertly tattooed that I am sure they would have been missed by even the best sleuth.

On the same woman, I also missed a pair of prosthetic breasts that were so expertly reconstructed that I could hardly find a scar (apparently the cosmetic surgeons had gone through the belly button and armpits, and reconstructed both breasts). The fact that I had missed that the deceased had tattooed eyebrows and fake breasts caused a huge stir.

The lawyer then went on to discredit me in the witness box, saying that I had performed the autopsy on the wrong body! I was incensed by this (false) accusation. The lawyer had managed to create so much doubt in the cross-examination that months went by and lots of money was spent before the trial finally ended. The perpetrator ended up getting a lighter sentence.

If you ask me, we need to take the politics out of science and put the science back into politics. We should also get doctors out of the courts and lawyers out of the hospitals, especially the so-called ambulance chasers.

15

On equality in death

'Coroner to the Stars' Thomas Tsunetomi Noguchi was the County of Los Angeles' chief medical examiner–coroner from 1967 to 1982. He garnered fame through high-profile cases such as the autopsies on John Belushi, Sharon Tate, Robert F. Kennedy and Marilyn Monroe. How does one perform a medicolegal autopsy on a Michael Jackson, an Amy Winehouse, or the president of a country? The correct answer: in exactly the same way as you would on any poor, helpless, defenceless or homeless person.

After all, it could happen that the famous person could die and arrive at the mortuary as a John Doe or Jane Doe. Often, the identity of the deceased is only established later. This means the autopsy has to be conducted at the same standard for all. On the face of it, we are all equal in death.

However, it is also true that not all medicolegal facilities have whole-body CT with 3D reconstruction and volume rendering, X-ray facilities, post-mortem CT angiography, post-mortem magnetic resonance tomography or post-mortem magnetic resonance angiography. Furthermore, not all facilities have state-of-the-art forensic toxicology facilities.

Take, for example, the latest medicolegal laboratories in the

USA, which cost approximately $95 million to build. In one such a facility's underground parking area, you'll find concrete support pillars surrounded by copper pipes that are connected to a refrigeration unit. This is so that, should there ever be a mass disaster in that region, the parking lot can be transformed into a massive, working cold room. Also, surrounding each concrete pillar is a pipe that supplies boiling water, so that the medical examiners or forensic pathologists can make tea or coffee while they work. Is this not forward thinking?

Patricia Cornwell – the best-selling crime writer and creator of the character Kay Scarpetta, a medical examiner – donated the money for what is known as Scarpetta House at this particular facility, a large room designed to give future forensic investigators a space to practise their crime scene analysis skills.[51] The house is complete with a living room, kitchen and bedroom. The death scene simulation exercises here may be compared to a state-of-the-art flight simulator for the latest jet airliner.

However, there are many places on the African continent with no medicolegal laboratories. If you die in some parts, no one will even pick up your body. I have heard of people who have literally become roadkill, with scavengers pecking the compressed human remains off the gravel road.

What would happen if one of your loved ones were to die on holiday in a developing country? Would you be able to rely on their forensic authorities to perform the best possible medicolegal examination and post-mortem, and discover the true cause of his or her death?

Many developing countries have no formal medicolegal system in place. In fact, as mentioned earlier there have been cases of forensic experts simply disappearing when they find something at autopsy that inadvertently implicated the authorities. So, if you think we are not equal in life, wait until death. Is this fair? Is this just?

I believe a country should be measured by how it treats its dead, and also by how it treats its medicolegal fatalities.

Ideally, a country should have six forensic pathologists per million people. In some African countries, there are no forensic pathologists whatsoever. In other African countries there is less than one forensic pathologist per million people. This will most likely result in burnout of the forensic pathologists concerned, and a lowering of the medicolegal standards. South Africa, for example, needs at least 150 forensic pathologists to function adequately, but currently has only 56. Three hundred forensic pathologists would be paradise.

The bioethical principle of distributive justice concerns the common good and the socially just allocation of goods in a society. The concept of justice is based on the assumption of the equal worth of all persons. Distributive justice is all about the fairness in how rights or resources are distributed. It refers to the perceived fairness of one's outcomes. With the amount of money needed to perform one heart transplant, a million immunisations can be done. How does this equation translate to forensics and the medicolegal examination of death, specifically on the African continent?

Can good medicine and good forensic science still be practised with limited resources? After all, distributive justice only becomes an issue when there is scarcity. Cost containment, also called resource allocation, is a euphemism for rationing. Can one practise good forensic medicine without X-rays, CTs,

MRIs or a functioning toxicology laboratory?

Forensic systems were developed when there were fewer people on the planet, but today we suffer from the massive burden of overpopulation. This means limited space and limited resources. It also brings a greater burden of unnatural deaths. How does one provide state-of-the-art autopsies to an ever-growing population, and with little or no money?

Distributive justice asks the question of how the financial pie is divided. Theoretically, each person could receive an equal share. Or, each person could receive a share according to how much he or she needs, or contributed to the pie, or merits a share of the pie. After many years of pondering this question, I believe the best answer is to be found in blockchain technology. By design, blockchain is a decentralised technology – the blockchain is a shared public ledger on which the entire pie-division network will rely.

Modern society is so complex that humans simply cannot manage the division of the pie themselves. Algorithms, therefore, offer the best possible way to do so. For example, I would not eat the crust of the pie (because I am currently on a low-carb diet), so you are welcome to the crust and you might give me some of the meat. The vegetarian may eat only the vegetables of the pie. Blockchain technology algorithms will probably be the cornerstone of the future of health economics.

What is the best way to bring a state-of-the-art forensic system and a first-class medicolegal service to poor and resource-strapped countries? My provisional answer is that this is indeed possible, when government and society pull together. This could entail privatisation or public–private partnerships. Forensics could be nationalised or practised independently if certain arms of government were privatised. Remember, the whole of society benefits from a good medicolegal system. The profession also needs better marketing to attract more people into the workforce.

Perhaps an even more controversial solution could be found in the concept of the humble hamburger. If commercial hamburger franchises can enter lower-income markets and succeed, then surely a system of forensic medical examiners can enter any marketplace and succeed. If we can industrialise the hamburger, then surely we can industrialise the medicolegal investigation of an unnatural death?

This chapter started with the question, 'Are we all equal in death?' I would like to counter that with the following question: 'Are we all equal in life?'

Earlier, I briefly mentioned the concept of luck egalitarianism. According to this view, some people are in their current situation because of brute luck (for example, through misfortunes in genetic makeup) and some people are in their current situation due to the consequences of conscious choices. Who would you feel more sorry for – the child with the genetic abnormality or the adult who drank too much alcohol and abused drugs? As a medical practitioner, would you treat these two patients equally? If resources are limited, why waste money on the self-destructive person?

Now let us take this one step further. Imagine that you are a trauma surgeon and two patients are brought to your casualty department at the same time. The history, as obtained from the ambulance staff, is as follows: one is a hijacker and the other is an off-duty policeman. Both have sustained gunshot wounds and are unconscious.

Who is the good guy, and who is the bad guy?

Would you be able to treat the two patients in exactly the same way? Would you be judgemental in any way? Who would you treat first, especially if you were the only trauma surgeon on duty? What happens if the hijacker has worse injuries than the off-duty policeman? Protocol demands that you treat the most severely injured person first.

The doctor is the doctor, and not the judge.

Now, what if the off-duty policeman was actually the hijacker? Only a court of law could realistically determine the ultimate truth. By judging, you assume that the hijacker is guilty, but nothing has been proven yet.

This is why it is the duty of a healthcare professional to provide care without fear, favour or judgement. Imagine how difficult this may be if you know you are treating a murderer, rapist, or hijacker.

If a person gets killed by the police, the law demands that the medicolegal investigation be observed by the Independent Police Investigative Directorate (IPID), the local criminal record centre, detectives, photographers, etc. When this happens, the mortuary literally swarms with people and I can hardly move. The reasons stem from human rights abuses in the past; I fully understand and appreciate this.

However, when a police officer is killed by a criminal, it is typically just me and the deceased in the mortuary. To me, this does not seem fair or just. Sometimes special task teams are set up for certain types of cases, but not for others. Why is one injustice worse (to you) than another injustice? These are some of the other kinds of inequalities in death.

The public always wants to know the grisly details of the

autopsy on a famous actor or high-profile individual. They rarely want to know about the autopsy on John Doe or Jane Doe. What if I were to tell you that we have autopsied people who were unidentified at the time and seemed destitute, and who later turned out to be very important in the eyes of the public?

It also concerns me that medical students and detectives often say that they do not want to attend an autopsy on a child, since they find it too traumatic. They say they would more easily attend the autopsy of an elderly person. I cannot make sense of this argument. A human being is a human being, irrespective of age. Does this mean that you would treat the elderly person with less care, emotion and respect than the child? Surely not.

Are we really all equal in death?

What about when a colleague takes great pride in the fact that he or she performed the autopsy on a celebrity? The autopsy of a celebrity should be performed to the same standard as the autopsy on a beggar.

This, at least, is how I approach my work. I try to do the best possible autopsy on every single body that ends up on my autopsy table. Forensically, we are all equal in death.

16

The Lindy Effect and forensics

If something has happened before, it will most likely happen again in the future. This insight has been proven time and again during my career as a forensic pathologist, and can be very helpful. It has even been described in academic literature; it is called the Lindy Effect.

In his book *Skin in the Game*, N.N. Taleb explains that the Lindy Effect got its name from a deli in New York, called Lindy's, which was famous for its cheesecake and all the actors who went there. Taleb writes:

> [B]ut in fact has been known for fifty or so years by physicists and mathematicians thanks to the heuristic that developed there. Actors who hung out there gossiping about other actors discovered that Broadway shows that lasted for, say, one hundred days, had a future life expectancy of one hundred more. For those that lasted two hundred days, two hundred more.
>
> The heuristic became known as the Lindy effect. A book that has been a hundred years in print is likely to stay in print another hundred years.[52]

The Lindy Effect is a theory that the future life expectancy of certain non-perishable things is proportional to their current age, so that every additional period of survival implies a longer remaining life expectancy. If one really looks at the mathematical principle behind this heuristic, one can see its effect in forensics as well. According to the Lindy Effect, we can usually expect more of the same to happen. The best predictor of future behaviour is past behaviour. If you hire someone who has changed jobs five times in the past five years, chances are pretty good that they will change jobs again within the next five years. What this means in terms of forensic pathology is that people with criminal records are most likely to commit further crimes in the future. If someone tried unsuccessfully to commit suicide in the past, they will most likely try to commit suicide again in the future.

The Lindy Effect also has sociopolitical implications. The fact that people will generally continue to do what they have been doing, and doing something they are comfortable with, means that they are unlikely to change radically. People like their routines and habits, and generally prefer stability.

Imagine taking a muffin tray and throwing glass marbles on top of it. Most of the marbles will settle into the muffin cups; others will end up resting on the tray surface. There are now two options: either you can wait for a prolonged period to see whether some of the marbles will eventually roll into the muffin cups, or you can shake the muffin tray to force the marbles into the muffin cups. Of course, having all of the marbles inside the muffin cups represents the more stable situation.

My muffin tray and marble analogy alludes to thermodynamics and equilibrium states. Sometimes a large amount of energy must be injected into a system for it to become more stable. In metallurgy and materials science, for example, you will encounter the term 'annealing'. This is a heat treatment that alters the physical and chemical properties of a material so that the material progresses towards its equilibrium state. What this means is that you have injected a large amount of energy into a system and made it stronger and more stable.

The Lindy Effect is essentially a heuristic about behaviour and the patterns of people's daily lives. What does this mean for forensics and medicine in general? If one gets a drunken male patient in the ER who sustained a stab wound on a Friday night at a party from getting into some or other altercation, chances are that he will present at the ER again, on an unspecified future date, with another drunken-altercation-related stab wound. This person's *pattern* could be such that his risks of being stabbed in the drunken state are greater than that of the general population.

If you can identify the patterns in your or another person's life, you could perhaps intervene and make a difference by disrupting the pattern. Disrupting patterns will require injecting a vast amount of energy, though, and it will be inconvenient.

If you combine the Lindy Effect with years of practising as a forensic pathologist, you will realise that some relationship advice could be gleaned from the autopsy table. Often, certain physical signs – or a combination of them – on someone's external body will tell you something about the kind of person you are dealing with. You will recall that we discussed Locard's principle of interchange earlier – every contact leaves a trace. Well, even your lifestyle will leave a trace on you. And if you can identify these traces, you will be able to make inferences about people from the traces left on them. These traces may be *overt* (such as needle track marks on their arms) or *covert* (such as certain behavioural changes).

At this point, I need to insert a disclaimer: there is no absolute statistical relationship between these external physical signs and the forensic manner of death. All I am saying is that many of the unnatural deaths I have examined over the years tend to be associated with certain signs. So, if person A died an unnatural death and showed one of these signs, then one of these signs could be associated with a risk of dying an unnatural death. Ergo, if A = B and B = C, then A = C.

My reasoning is as follows: since many of the bodies on the autopsy table tend to show some of the following physical signs, you might do well to heed the following practical relationship advice.

Scars and needle puncture marks: If you are on a date and notice multiple scars on your date's body, there is a good chance that the scars are from repeated fighting or previous accidents. If he or she has been in fights before, there is a great likelihood, according to the Lindy Effect that there will be more fights or accidents in the future. Cubital fossa scars from multiple needle punctures could indicate a history of intravenous drug abuse. If there are multiple, parallel, tentative incision scars on the ventral aspect of his or her less dominant wrist, it could point to previous suicide attempts.

Obviously, there are many reasons for scars and one cannot jump to conclusions, but generally speaking, scars of this nature should raise some questions in your mind.

Tattoos: Tattoos have become very popular in recent decades. Of course, there is a huge difference between fashion tattoos and what I call 'danger' tattoos: those received in prison, for example. Tattoos of animals, general objects and symbols are quite common and don't generally point to anything, but beware of gang-related tattoos and tattoos on the face, neck or hands. The 26s, 27s and 28s are well-known gangs in South Africa. An RAF 4 tattoo on the front of the lower leg indicates that the person has escaped from prison. RAF stands for Royal Air Force, which in a prison context refers to something completely different.

When you enter a certain criminal culture or subculture, that culture tends to leave its Locard's mark on you. For example, certain gangs tattoo themselves on the inner aspect of their lower lip.

Other forms of body art: Of the strangest things I have seen in the past decade or so, specifically on prisoners and ex-prisoners, are multiple subcutaneous penile beads. Small incisions are apparently made on the shaft of the penis, and glass beads are inserted under the skin. This makes the penis look rather like a Lunch Bar.

Signs of chronic bad health: Epitrochlear lymph nodes (fleshy lymph nodes on the inner aspects of the elbows), candida (thrush) on the mouth, bilateral temporal or masseter muscle wasting (where you can see the cheek bones very easily), chronic wasting disease, rashes or bad skin, bad dental hygiene, halitosis (bad breath) and an emaciated body are physical signs that have been associated with certain kinds of forensic cases.

So, if you're sitting with someone who is chain-smoking, looks somewhat agitated and tends to touch their nose every now and again, chances are good that they have a history of using psychostimulants. There is also a chance of underlying bipolar mood disorder and/or masked depression. It is also likely that the person has an addictive personality type. There is, however, a small chance that they may simply be suffering from hayfever or allergies.

Therefore, do not enter a committed relationship with any-one until you can answer the following four questions, at least, about that person:

1. How does he or she act when drunk? The English writer Thomas De Quincey wrote, 'Sobriety disguiseth man!' If you want to know who your partner is, get him or her drunk and the real person will shine through.

2. How does he or she act when angry? The American writer and orator Robert Green Ingersoll wrote, 'Anger is a wind which blows out the lamp of the mind.'

3. What does he or she spend money on? Does he or she spend it on drugs, prostitutes or gambling? Personally, I would rather spend my time with a low-income person with much class than with a high-income person with little class.

4. How does he or she spend his or her leisure time? Is free time spent on meaningful hobbies or untoward activities?

It is said that pretence disappears in situations involving money, in moments of anger, or in the way a man takes his liquor.[53] Once you can confidently answer these four questions in a positive way, you should be safe to embark on a relationship.

17

Ten lessons for the living from the dead

What can the dead teach us, the living? After performing thousands of autopsies, I have distilled ten lessons from the autopsy table.

1. Do not tempt fate

A female leopard gives birth to two cubs. One cub is brave and adventurous, while the other is cautious and hesitant. As in nature, I believe there are also brave cubs and safe cubs in the human world. The brave cubs are the go-getters, the explorers, the adventurers; they are consequently more exposed to risk. The safe cubs are more averse to risk.

While the brave cubs tempt fate, the safe cubs do not. There are those in this world who wake up and tempt fate. They often work in high-risk jobs; some even prefer to take their holidays in unsafe destinations. From a forensic point of view, I would argue that one is probably better off being a safe cub.

I am often asked what tempting fate entails. Well, as we all know some neighbourhoods are more dangerous than others. By walking alone at night through a dangerous neighbourhood, you are tempting fate. You would also be tempting fate by being outdoors in a thunderstorm. It is all a matter of risk and risk awareness.

I once received an e-mail from a British tourist who had gone on a safari in Namibia with his wife. The safari had been arranged by a tour company. On one of the days, they were in an open-top overland vehicle watching leopards mating when an electrical thunderstorm unleashed itself. Half the tour group wanted to watch the leopards in the rain. The other half wanted to get back safely to camp.

The tourist asked what his risk of being hit by lightning would have been. Furthermore, he wanted to know whether he could take legal action against the tour company. I responded with my dangerous neighbourhood metaphor and by repeating my mantra to go indoors when thunder roars. I believed, in this instance, that the tour guide was tempting fate. The prudent thing to have done would have been to head back to camp immediately.

The reasonable tour guide test should have been applied. What would a reasonable tour guide have done, in similar situation, anywhere else on earth? Does the tour company have protocols and standard operating procedures for such an eventuality?

What are the actual risks of getting struck by lightning, sitting in an open-top overland vehicle, in Africa, during an electrical thunderstorm? If you crunched the numbers and looked at the statistics, you would soon find out that the odds of being struck by lightning are greater outdoors than indoors.

Yes, the tourists paid a lot of money to travel to Namibia and by all accounts this was a very special sighting. One can imagine the irate guests who, upon seeing mating leopards for the first time in their lives, were forced to head back to camp because of a light drizzle and the possibility of thunder and lightning.

This is not a black-and-white situation, but the inconvenience of missing a rare leopard sighting would be less than the inconvenience of a vehicle-load full of dead and lightning-injured tourists.

2. Do not live recklessly

Keep yourself and your loved ones safe. You will know when you are being reckless. Trust your gut.

From a forensic point of view, I see people go off the rails from time to time. This is okay, provided you stay parallel to the railway tracks. If you begin to travel perpendicular to the railway tracks, however, it is not good.

Feeling unsure and lost? Try to remember that this is part of life. Take a breath, you'll be okay.

Do what you need to do to make yourself happy, but do it in a responsible way.

There are plot points in every person's life – points where something happens or is caused to happen that changes the direction and circumstances of your existence. You need to have the insight and foresight to realise when you hit the bad plot points in your life. For example, you will most likely become like the people with whom you spend the most time. Choose your friends wisely and carefully.

Also keep in mind that life's thunderstorms come and go. When you no longer know what to do, you might find that your real journey has just begun. Be safe during the emotional thunderstorm. Once it has passed, there will be peace.

There are things which you are in charge of, such as your actions, your emotions, your mood state, your behaviour, your efforts, your ideas, your beliefs and your motivation.

Sadly, you have no control over other things, such as what others think of you, what they feel about you, their actions towards you, how they talk to you, or their judgements of you.

I think that the most important way forward is to answer quietly the personal question of where your contribution in life lies, and then to work tirelessly towards that contribution.

3. Do not travel too fast

I have witnessed so many unnecessary motor vehicle accident deaths. People often misjudge their speed. When I am driving and a car speeds past I think, *What is the rush?* Do people not understand the risks to which they are exposing themselves?

I also know so many people who dream of owning a motorbike. The motorbike has been romanticised since the days of James Dean. The truth of the matter is that motorbikes are very dangerous. Some people, especially those who are young and full of testosterone, should simply not own motorbikes. I have performed too many autopsies on motorbike-related deaths.

But try having this conversation with people. You will not win. Some of the smartest people I know own motorbikes and are speed freaks. You often find that these same people call those who travel slower than them fools, and those who travel faster than them idiots!

Traffic accidents can be caused by a variety of things, including weather conditions, the condition of the vehicle or the road, or reasons relating to the driver. The person behind the wheel could have a heart attack or a stroke, or may fall asleep at the wheel. People also have accidents because they type text messages while driving, or they hit animals that are crossing the road. Still, the most common cause of death in motor vehicle accidents is speeding.

My humble advice is to leave earlier and travel slower. Enjoy the scenery and observe the sights around you.

4. Pick the right partner

When you are about to choose a life partner, pick one who will be good for you as a person. It's not important that he or she is good for your parents, your bank account or your image. Choose someone who is going to enrich your life.

If you choose the wrong partner and let the wrong people into your life, joy, peace, love and hope will go missing from your life. However, your life will be filled with all these things if you can find someone who wants to listen to you, learn from you and see you win, and who supports your vision.

Try to find a partner who is honest and straightforward. Try to find a partner who is kind. The resulting lack of drama makes life so much easier. A perfect relationship does not mean that you will never get angry, upset or irritated with each other. It's about how quickly you can resolve conflict and bounce back to normal. Beware people who keep on fighting and who do not want peace. It is best to walk away from them.

I often refer to the architecture metaphor – if the walls of a relationship are cracked, no amount of wallpaper will solve the problem. Fix the cracks. Also, you need a strong and solid foundation in order to build a tall building. You start building from the ground upwards, not from the top downwards.

Don't waste your time on a partner or friends who don't appreciate you. Do not trust someone who has let you down more than twice. Once was a warning. Twice was a lesson. Anything more than that is simply taking advantage. Remember the Lindy Effect.

There are people who will build you up and people who will tear you down. But in the end, you'll thank them both. You owe your loyalty to those who never made you question theirs.

There are four main mathematical symbols (addition, subtraction, multiplication and division). Be with those who add and multiply and avoid those who subtract and divide. Go where you are celebrated, not tolerated. Be with those who make you feel good about yourself and not those who make you doubt yourself.

Stay away from people who can't take responsibility for their actions.

Walk away from arguments that lead you to anger and from any thought that undermines your peace of mind. Walk away from those who will never see your worth.

Walk away from people who poison your soul.

5. Do not overindulge

Everyone needs to choose one of two pains in life: the pain of discipline or the pain of regret. It may be okay to indulge once in a while, but be careful of overindulging. Sadly, far too often overindulgence is a cause of unnatural death.

Yes, we all get distracted in life. Sometimes, these distractions are healthy (a good book, a movie, or company, for example). However, many other distractions are unhealthy.

Try to starve your unhealthy distractions and feed your positive distractions. Always ask yourself whether what you are doing right now is:

1. natural and necessary
2. natural and unnecessary
3. unnatural and unnecessary.

People mostly overindulge in smoking or alcohol. Some people overindulge in eating junk food and bad carbohydrates. Others overindulge in using recreational drugs. Some people overindulge with work. 'Karoshi' is a Japanese term that can be translated literally as 'overwork death'. It is also known as occupational sudden mortality. The major medical causes of karoshi deaths are heart attack and stroke due to stress. The first case of karoshi was reported in 1969 when a twenty-nine-year-old male worker at Japan's largest newspaper company had a stroke. The term was invented in 1978 to refer to an increasing number of people suffering from fatal strokes and heart attacks attributed to overwork.

Nothing in life is *that* important. Remember, they don't write accolades on a tombstone – they write, 'In loving memory of family, and children.' It will always be the people in your life who matter most. It is they who should be your greatest indulgence.

6. Avoid doing stupid things

The Darwin Awards have been bestowed in a tongue-in-cheek manner since 1985. According to the website for the awards: 'In the spirit of Charles Darwin, the Darwin Awards commemorate individuals who protect our gene pool by making the ultimate sacrifice of their own lives. Darwin Award winners eliminate themselves in an extraordinarily idiotic manner, thereby improving our species' chances of long-term survival.'

Accidental self-sterilisation also qualifies; however, the website notes: 'Of necessity, the award is usually bestowed posthumously.' The candidate is disqualified, though, if innocent bystanders, who might have contributed positively to the gene pool, are killed in the process.

I'm afraid to say that I have seen a few potential Darwin Award candidates end up on my autopsy table. Take, for example, the man who accidentally shot himself while innocently demonstrating the use of a firearm to a friend. This happens more often than you'd think.

There have been accidental deaths due to electrocution during amateur electro-fishing. Electro-fishing (passing electricity through water to catch fish) requires sophisticated equipment. Crude and illegal forms of electro-fishing are used from time to time; ever so often, people get electrocuted. There are case reports of accidental electrocution deaths while fishing in waterlogged fields using electricity drawn from overhead lines.[54]

7. Be more mindful

It is part of our DNA as *Homo sapiens* to complain. In some instances, complaining about something that's wrong can help to raise awareness about a problem. It can even help to make the problem go away – and to make the whole system better for everyone.

It is important, though, to be mindful of yourself and those around you.

Being more mindful implies thinking more carefully about what you are doing and how you are doing it. It requires that you do not react viscerally (respond automatically without thinking about the consequences).

I have seen incredibly bad consequences of the actions of people who were not mindful and who said the wrong thing in front of the wrong people, in the wrong place, in the wrong context or at the wrong time. The text you write in anger. The e-mail you send without considering the aftermath. These may cause untold damage to you and the ones you love.

It takes about twenty years to build a reputation, and about five minutes to destroy it.

Fortunately, forensics tends to engender mindfulness. It also helps develop mental toughness. To be mentally strong, you have to monitor your emotions. If you work on yourself, I believe that the rest will follow.

My colleagues and I meet over a cup of tea or coffee every morning. We try to monitor our emotions throughout the day and recognise how our feelings influence our thoughts and our behaviours. You have to try to be realistically optimistic – that is, try to be kind to yourself and to your colleagues, manage your time wisely, focus on productive activities, strive to fulfil your purpose and try to focus on the bigger picture. Try to do the right thing. I find that this makes others more appreciative of what we do.

The power of positive reinforcement cannot be understated. Animal trainers can train animals to do incredible things with positive reinforcement. I have seen birds fly around the room three times and through a hoop because of positive reinforcement. Negative reinforcement also works, yet it tends to breed animosity and resentment towards the animal trainer. It is a little-known fact, but many lion tamers ended up savaged and mauled by their own lions, despite their cracking whips.

You begin to understand that, like physically strong people need to train regularly to stay in good shape, you need to keep working your 'mental muscles' to prevent atrophy. Daily, you need to monitor your own progress, and always try to move forwards. You cannot always control what's happening around you, but you must challenge yourself to control the way in which you respond to it.

Be nicer to people, compliment them, and say 'good work' more often. This is where your power lies.

8. Care about yourself more

The world is such a crazy place, and so complex, that all you can do is live your own life.

You can also start each day by taking better care of yourself. I begin each day by taking five deep, slow breaths while I'm still lying in bed, then slowly getting out of bed.

Be more mindful of the cosmetics you wear, such as your makeup, perfume, or aftershave. Pathologists have located these in the digestive tract – most of these toxic chemicals you wear on your face just end up being transferred or swallowed during a normal day (remember Locard's principle). Some perfumes and aftershaves have prolonged half-lives. A perfume may cling to an object for a prolonged period – forensic experts have even used cosmetic transfer to catch criminals.[55]

I have found that in many male suicide cases, the men are unshaven. In *Man's Search for Meaning*, Holocaust survivor

Victor Frankl wrote that he could predict who was going to die based on who was no longer looking after themselves. 'Everything can be taken from a man but one thing: the last of human freedoms – to choose one's attitude in any given set of circumstances, to choose one's own way.'[56]

Back in the day, when I was a clinical doctor, I instinctively knew when a patient was ready for discharge from the hospital – they would begin to take better care of themselves. They were sufficiently healed to begin to care about the way they looked. Their scalp hair was neat, for example.

Appreciate every single person who has tried to brighten your days, even if it's just with a short message to ask if you're okay. It is the little things that matter most.

Be kind to yourself. You are not an inexhaustible resource.

9. Care about others more

If you want to depress yourself, go to any mortuary in South Africa on a Monday morning and station yourself by the telephone. You will hear the phone ring multiple times. The calls are typically the same: people looking for their lost loved ones.

The missing person had usually gone out on Friday or Saturday night, and had not yet returned home. It astounds me how many people do not tell their families where they are going or what time they will be back home. These people do not seem to care about others.

It is scary to think that one day you're going to have to live without your mother or father or brother or sister or husband or wife or best friend. Appreciate your loved ones while you can; none of us is going to be here forever.

You do not have to be a medical doctor to save someone's

life. All you have to do is be aware of those around you. The most precious gift you can give is your time and attention, so be kind to others. If kindness is the easiest gift to give, why is it so hard to find? Nothing you do makes any sense if you don't touch the hearts of others.

It is not what you do once in a while that shapes your life – it is what you do every day.

There are two types of death. The first type of death is when you physically die and the second type of death is when those who are dear to you totally forget about you. You have minimal control over the first type of death. You do, however, have a lot of control over the second type of death. You can accelerate or retard the second type of death by what you are doing right now, while you are still alive. People lead ever-lonelier lives on an increasingly connected planet.

If the world is hurtling through space, bound eventually to evaporate when our sun expands and explodes, then human history is a directionless romp through time, you and I are going nowhere, and life has no significance. Why work, why build, why love, if it all ends in nothingness? Why even care?

The world may have no purpose – or it may have a purpose. No one knows for certain. We are all here, on this rock, right now, at this specific point in time. Therefore, let us all try to make our time here somewhat pleasant for one another.

Earlier, I mentioned that it astounds me just how many people have no support system and how it would always be the landlord or cleaner who finds the decomposed body in the apartment, and never a family member. Try to get to know your neighbours and check up on them regularly. From time to time, phone old friends and invite them for tea, coffee or a milkshake. Embrace the transience of things. Enjoy your loved ones, your friends, your pets and your community. Enjoy the flowers while they last!

10. Be humble – or, at least, don't be arrogant!

Some people are congenitally arrogant, and do not even realise how arrogant they are. These people usually have incredibly thick skins and don't mind trampling on others. These people are usually the older versions of the brave cubs.

It is one of the great tragedies in life that too many people are taken in by character, and too few by wisdom or knowledge. Those who study are often so busy reading that they tend to neglect their character. And those who are busy developing their character on the streets don't have any time to read. So we end up being inspired by fools with great character!

If you are arrogant in forensics, you sign your own professional death warrant. You cannot and may not be arrogant in this field. Every day, you are humbled by what you see.

If you are arrogant or dogmatic in court, you will see your backside. I have seen mighty forensic pathologists with over forty years of experience crumble in court. In this field, you seldom say 'never' and 'always'.[57] There are only seven answers that a forensic pathologist will ever give in a court of law:

1. Certainly not.
2. Very likely not.
3. Likely not.
4. 50/50.
5. Likely was.
6. Very likely was.
7. Certainly was.

To give an exact number or an exact percentage of a particular event occurring would also be to commit professional suicide.

By way of example, if the prosecution asked me, 'What are the chances of the deceased's head injury being caused by a brick?' I would answer, 'Very likely,' but I would never answer with a specific figure or percentage.

Humility has stood me in relatively good stead in my professional life. If I do not know the answer, I say that I do not know, that I will have to consult a more senior colleague or research the answer. For this reason, I encourage people to try to be more humble – or, at least, to be less arrogant.

18

On death and dying

As a forensic pathologist I deal not only with the dead but also with the living, especially at the scene of death and in the mortuary when family members come to identify a body. I usually see the following reactions among those who have lost a loved one: shock and disbelief; anger; guilt and blame; sorrow and depression; and, eventually, acceptance.

One of my forensic heroes is the late Dr Lester Adelson, a pre-eminent American forensic pathologist who was instrumental in the development and refinement of forensic pathology.[58] He once said, 'Regardless of colour, race, sex, or the shape of the nose, everyone has the same red blood at autopsy, and tears that are shed for a lost loved one are equally salty.'[59]

To reach a point of acceptance, it is necessary to go through all the phases of grief. It is important to understand that anger, shock, feelings of guilt and even denial may just be an expression of sorrow and bereavement, and should never be taken personally. All these stages are considered to be normal reactions.

It is not advisable to take tranquilisers or alcohol to suppress these normal human bereavement processes. A bereavement becomes abnormal when it lasts abnormally long, when it starts to affect your normal life, and when sorrow cannot be resolved into the late stage of acceptance. It is always important to monitor your own and your loved ones' reactions to death. If your emotions become too much to handle, it is best to seek out a professional bereavement counsellor.

Over the years, I have seen some extreme cases of bereavement and mourning. There was, for example, a case of a severely emotionally traumatised relative who pulled out his gun at the mortuary and started shooting out of some of the windows.

On the other end of the spectrum, we have had Oscar-winning cases of faked bereavement. In one instance, several individuals come to the mortuary and wailed dramatically over the coffin of the deceased. After a thorough investigation, it proved to be a case of fraud: the wailers had in fact murdered the deceased to claim his life insurance. They were part of a syndicate who had killed the person and then pretended to be family and friends.

In another case, a family member was incredibly overenthusiastic at a death scene and tried everything in his power to help with our investigation. It later transpired that he was in fact the murderer. To quote Lester again, 'In the autopsy room, we see people with their naked bodies; when families see us, we see their guilt, grief, and greed; we see families with their naked souls.'[60]

It is a sad reality that criminals prey on people when they are at their weakest and most vulnerable. No other industry has such potential for corruption than the death industry. I have encountered several scams surrounding death. One crafty conman phoned a mourning widow to sympathise about her husband's death and pretended to be a carpet dealer. He told her that her husband had purchased an expensive Persian rug for her before his death. 'We want to deliver it to you, but we don't know where to deliver it. He bought it as a gift for you before his death. He still owes us several thousand on the payment. What do we do?' he asked her.

The Persian carpet salesman had read about her husband's death in the obituary column of the newspaper and cold-called her.

The spectrum of forensic pathology seen in Africa seems richer and more varied than elsewhere. Besides the great weather and the great people, Africa forces you to live through your senses. It is paradise for a forensic pathologist. While my job might entail dealing with death all day long, no other field highlights the concepts of resilience and fragility quite like forensics.

The following story illustrates the remarkable healing and regenerative powers of the human body. It is from the time when I was working as a general practitioner in Phalaborwa. A man who had been living on the tribal lands for quite some time and didn't seem very exposed to the trappings of the western world came to the hospital.

When he shook my hand, his palm felt like leather. He had one of the toughest, strongest, biggest hands I had ever seen. He could not speak English; I had to ask a local nursing sister to translate for me.

Apparently, the man had fractured his tibia and fibula (sustained a right lower leg fracture). An external fixator (a type of metallic rod that is screwed into bone to stabilise a fracture on the outside of the body) had been applied by the local orthopaedic surgeon. What surprised me was that this had happened six years earlier.

Instead of coming back to see the doctor for removal in six weeks, he had somehow heard that he had to wait six years! He had been walking around with an external fixator for *six years*.

After much surprise and disbelief we removed the external fixator, and the wounds had healed beautifully. There were no signs of infection; the bones had knitted perfectly.

Given the right conditions, all wounds will heal – the human body can be incredibly robust, anti-fragile and resilient. Obviously, wounds will not heal if the conditions are not right (for example, if one has background diabetes mellitus). However, a fit, healthy person, eating a healthy, natural diet, exposed to sunshine and water and the elements will, as a rule, heal perfectly.

I have also seen humans survive being shot multiple times. At times the human body seems very resilient – but at other times, very fragile. I have seen people who had been punched on the head or the chest die immediately. For example, a person who has osteogenesis imperfecta, also known as brittle bone syndrome, is more likely to be injured or die from a punch to the head than a person from the general population.

Sometimes, the smallest amount of blunt force trauma to the head can kill. This is often the case with people suffering from eggshell skull syndrome. Interestingly, in criminal law the maxim is that the defendant must 'take their victims as they find them' – therefore, the frailty, weakness or feebleness of a victim cannot be used as a defence in court.

Another example would be commotio cordis, or agitation of the heart. This is a disruption of heart rhythm that occurs as a result of a blow to the area directly over the heart at a critical time during the cycle of a heartbeat. It causes cardiac arrest. Sudden unexpected cardiac death that occurs in young people during sports participation is usually associated with previously diagnosed or undiagnosed structural or electrical cardiac abnormalities. Sometimes, the smallest amount of blunt force trauma to the front of the chest can kill a person.

The brutal, messy truth is that no one really knows how resilient or fragile they are until the critical moment comes. I have seen the fittest special forces soldiers die in the prime of their lives from an underlying natural disease condition. I have also seen morbidly obese smokers and alcoholics live to ripe old ages, and die from a totally unrelated unnatural death.

On one of my autopsy tables lies a twenty-eight-year-old male with 75 per cent narrowing of his coronary arteries from atherosclerosis and no other ascertainable cause of death, so I sign the cause of death as probably in keeping with that of coronary artery disease. On my other autopsy table lies a sixty-eight-year-old male with 95 per cent narrowing of his coronary arteries from atherosclerosis (the coronary arteries are so obstructed that they appear to have pinpoint lumens to supply blood to the heart) who died from a homicidal gunshot wound to the head. I sign the cause of death as 'gun-shot to head'.

I cannot help but become philosophical when I see these kinds of cardiovascular pathologies. Why did the younger man who had relatively open coronary arteries die from his apparent heart condition, yet the older man with near-complete occlusion of his coronary arteries survived his?

I am very concerned about the way most people die in hospitals. The nursing sisters think that the doctors will talk to the patients and the doctors expect that the nursing sisters will talk to the patients. Often, no one is talking to the patients, and they die alone.

Some medical facilities practise what is called death rehearsal. Death rehearsal is a technique developed to help terminally ill patients and their families deal with anxieties about death. This entails asking the dying patient questions such as, 'Who do you think will attend your funeral, and who will not?', 'Do you have any regrets in your life?', 'Is there someone you need to make peace with before you die?' and 'Is there anyone to whom you want to confess anything?'[61]

While it can be very tough, I do believe it is a good thing for doctors to try to have an honest conversation with people who are dying and try to connect with them. Of course, it is important to try to connect with them from their personal belief system. It is no use trying to connect with an atheist if you are a Christian, or with a Jewish person if you are a Catholic priest.

I often ask dying people, 'Do you remember what it was like before you were born?' They often look at me in stunned silence, before I respond with, 'That is most probably what it will be like after you are dead.'

The truth of the matter is that death is hidden from the living. The average person will see only one or two dead people in their entire lives. In this book, I have tried, unapologetically, to show the facts, and systematically approached death in a way that may seem very foreign to you – but its purpose is to help open the eyes of the living.

My hope is that, in reading this book, you will be affected in a positive way, that you will have had a glimpse into the psychological requirements of dealing with this kind of thing. Perhaps you will learn to love and live more prudently and to cherish your time on earth.

My wish is that this book will help to make you more aware and more mindful. As the American magician Teller, of Penn & Teller fame, said: 'Try that yourself sometime: Take something (or someone) you love, and – in your imagination – say goodbye forever right now. Grieve for a moment. Then feel the explosion of happiness that comes when you remind yourself you don't have to say goodbye. At least, not yet.'

We close the eyes of the dead, but the dead open the eyes of the living.[62] The most real thing in the world is human suffering. Some deaths are slow and painful. Other deaths are quick and painless. For some, life is too long. For others, it is too short.

Most people seem to be more afraid of loneliness than death. It is not uncommon to arrive at a death scene and find an elderly couple dead, lying next to each other. Oftentimes, this may be due to a 'suicide pact'– where an elderly couple decide to commit suicide together. There are, however, cases on record in which the life partner of a deceased person died on the spot upon discovering the body of their loved one. Takotsubo cardiomyopathy, also known as stress cardiomyopathy, is a type of non-ischaemic cardiomyopathy in which there is a sudden temporary weakening of the muscular portion of the heart. This weakening may be triggered by emotional stress, such as the death of a loved one, a break-up, a rejection by a partner or constant anxiety. The name comes from the Japanese word meaning 'octopus trap', because the left ventricle takes on a shape resembling a fishing pot. It is commonly known as 'broken heart syndrome'.

This reminds me of another quote by Dr Lester Adelson about life as a forensic pathologist: 'You don't become hardened to death; you become more sensitive to it.'[63]

The problem with constant exposure to death and dying is that you can lose track of what is a healthy, normal society. Sometimes, I have to remind myself that there are countries on this planet with no gun-related deaths. At other times, I have to pinch myself when I realise that in some countries there are no forensic pathologists, simply because there is no need for them.

This is why I say that, when you dedicate your life to forensic pathology practice in Africa, you have to interrogate your motives critically for doing so. You need to be physically, emotionally and psychologically fit for this kind of work. It means embracing a hard life and an exacting job. Forensic pathology is a calling, almost religious in nature. You sacrifice personal relationships and monetary success.

'You haven't failed until you quit,' Norman Vaughan once said. So you don't quit. You just keep going.

In my brief time as a forensic pathologist in Africa the attrition rate has been staggering. Many of my colleagues have left the field. Some have become anatomical pathologists, which typically draws a better salary. Others have immigrated to greener pastures, with fewer autopsies. Some have even left the field completely. One now packs shelves as an assistant in a grocery store in England.

You may end up suffering what is known as care fatigue or moral injury. The constant stream of unnatural deaths in Africa can definitely deplete your reserves to care; you simply feel too fatigued to do so.

Sometimes, all you can think about is surviving the moment. At times, I have been behind schedule but kept going because I knew I would always catch up. Your mind is wired, sometimes, and you have difficulty sleeping.

It is always a grind. Some days it feels like you are pedalling against 60 km/h winds, in and out of loose sand and ruts. On these days, pure willpower and discipline gets you through.

I recall doing the autopsy on a severely decomposed body in the peak of an African summer. The air conditioners were not working. I approached the body, and a swarm of blowflies took off. The buzz reminded me of Jurassic Park; it reverberated deep inside my soul.

Some days, you feel high on fatigue and adrenalin. Some of my colleagues look a little haggard, others look grizzled. On other days, you feel strong and at peace, although these days are few and far between.

Chatting and joking with colleagues helps a lot. Having a good support system and motivation helps. Sometimes the road is magical, and I am reminded about why I am in this profession. Often, I think of all my reasons for being here, and I call them out in my mind.

Despite an unceasing stream of publications extolling the value of post-mortem examination, the hospital autopsy rate continues to decline in the world and in Africa.[64] Managers would rather spend money on the living, even though the dead can help to save the living. Try to explain this concept to policy makers . . .

I predict that the autopsy will slowly start to disappear from society. Within the next thirty years or so, there will probably be no more autopsies as we know them. I suspect there will be a greater reliance on post-mortem non-invasive virtual autopsy with CT and MRI scans, artificial intelligence and algorithms.

I expect that, in future, bodies will be processed robotically on a conveyer belt of sorts. They will be scanned, X-rayed, CT'ed, MRI'ed, photographed, filmed and washed by machines. Core-guided biopsies will be performed under radiological guidance. Toxicology will be performed on site by means of robotic needle aspiration.

Some days, I worry that soon there may be no more need for the medieval process that is the autopsy examination. I fear the day when I might have to stand on a street corner with a cardboard sign: 'Will do autopsy for food'!

Acknowledgements

My sincerest gratitude to my publisher, Annie Olivier, for all her wisdom and perseverance since our first meeting in 2017, and to the staff at Jonathan Ball. Thanks to Eugene Ashton for inspiring this journey. Thanks to Angela Voges for the editing.

I would like to thank Nicholas Sergio Cocciuti, Ralph Milbrandt and Rob G. Wermuth for their contributions to this book.

Thank you to Annelize Nienaber, Ian McKechnie and Belinda Mosdell for proofreading the initial drafts of this book.

Thanks to Thomas Birkenbach, Tessa Stuart, Elmi de Pauw and Daniel Fisher from Walla Films, and Servaas Rossouw for the photographs.

Thanks to Nicole Ermacora and Linda Pretorius for the proofreading.

Thanks to my uncles Brian Blumenthal and Julius Preddy for their wise counsel.

Thanks to Sageren Aiyer, Gavin Kirk and Sibusiso Ntsele for their kind and insightful reviews.

Special thanks to my parents, Walter and Diane, for their unwavering support during this process.

Karen, thank you, you have been amazing!

Finally, to my forensics colleagues in South Africa and abroad, thank you for making all our lives that little bit safer.

Glossary

algor mortis: the gradual cooling of the body following death

antiretroviral: denoting or relating to a class of drugs that inhibit the activity of retroviruses such as HIV

baroreceptor: a receptor that is sensitive to changes in pressure

blockchain: a system in which a record of transactions made in bitcoin or another cryptocurrency is maintained across several computers that are linked in a peer-to-peer network

cadaveric spasm: a rare form of muscular stiffening that occurs at the moment of death and persists into the period of rigor mortis

commotio cordis: Latin for 'agitation of the heart', an often-lethal disruption of heart rhythm that occurs as a result of a blow to the area directly over the heart (the precordial region) at a critical time during the cycle of a heartbeat, producing what is termed an R-on-T phenomenon

COVID-19: a disease caused by a new strain of coronavirus, with 'CO' denoting 'corona', 'VI' denoting 'virus' and 'D' denoting 'disease', '19' refers to the year '2019'

craniotomy: the surgical removal of a portion of the skull

delirium tremens: a psychotic condition typical of withdrawal in chronic alcoholics, involving tremors, hallucinations, anxiety and disorientation

DNA: deoxyribonucleic acid, a self-replicating material present in nearly all living organisms as the main constituent of chromosomes; the carrier of genetic information

Dürck's granuloma: sometimes seen in malaria cases, an area of rarefied brain containing activated microglia/macrophages appearing at the site of a prior ring haemorrhage

dyadic death: a violent event in which an individual commits homicide and subsequently commits suicide within a few hours

electrocardiogram (ECG): a recording of the electrical activity of the heart; it is a simple, non-invasive procedure in which electrodes are placed on the skin of the chest and connected in a specific order to a machine that measures electrical activity all over the heart

formaldehyde: a colourless, pungent gas in solution made by oxidising methanol

hemozoin pigment: an iron-containing pigment that accumulates as cytoplasmic granules in malaria parasites and is a breakdown product of haemoglobin

hypothermia: the condition of having an abnormally (typically dangerously) low body temperature

hyperthermia: the condition of having a body temperature that is greatly above normal

lividity: the process through which the body's blood supply will stop moving after the heart has stopped pumping; displays as a dark-purple discolouration on the gravity-dependent aspects of the body and is also referred to as livor mortis or post-mortem hypostasis

Locard's principle: a principle which holds that the perpetrator of a crime will bring something into the crime scene and leave with something from it, and that both can be used as forensic evidence

Nissen fundoplication: a surgical procedure to treat gastro-esophageal reflux disease (GERD) and hiatal hernia

nyaope: a narcotic substance, typically comprising heroin, marijuana and other substances, smoked as a recreational drug in some parts of South Africa

Mantoux test: a test for immunity to tuberculosis using intradermal injection of tuberculin

Mees' lines: a change that occurs in the colour of the nail with no palpable ridges, typically described as white bands traversing the nail bed, running parallel to the lunula across the entire nail bed; this finding is indicative of arsenic, thallium or other heavy metal poisoning.

oculocaloric reflex: the caloric reflex test is a test of the vestibulo-ocular reflex that involves irrigating cold or warm water or air into the external auditory canal; a method developed by Róbert Bárány, who won a Nobel prize in 1914 for this discovery

omentum: a fold of peritoneum connecting the stomach with other abdominal organs

osteoblast: a cell that builds bone

osteoclast: a large multinucleate bone cell that absorbs bone tissue during growth and healing

phenotype: to determine the set of observable characteristics of an individual resulting from the interaction of its genotype with the environment

parasympathetic nervous system: the part of the involuntary nervous system that serves to slow the heart rate, increase intestinal and glandular activity, and relax the sphincter muscles; together with the sympathetic nervous system, it constitutes the autonomic nervous system

post-exposure prophylaxis: a method of preventing certain virus infections; it involves using a drug or vaccine taken very soon after a person may have been exposed to the virus

prosector: a person with the task of preparing organs for dissection or demonstration, usually in medical schools or hospitals; the act of prosecting differs from the act of eviscerating, where the organs of the body are surgically removed

putrefaction: the process of decay or rotting in a body or other organic matter

purging: discharge of fluid that may simulate antemortem haemorrhage; typically caused by passive regurgitation of stomach contents after death

rigor mortis: stiffening of the joints and muscles of a body a few hours after death, usually lasting from one to four days

sympathetic nervous system: a part of the nervous system that serves to accelerate the heart rate, constrict blood vessels and raise blood pressure; with the parasympathetic nervous system, it constitutes the autonomic nervous system

taweez: an amulet or locket containing certain verses or prayers. It is usually worn to protect from evil.

vita minima: a state of apparent death

Notes

1 Schwär, T.G., Loubser, J.D. & Olivier, J.A. (1988). *The Forensic ABC in Medical Practice: A practical guide.* Pretoria: Haum Educational Publishers, pp. 395–397.

2 Ibid.

3 Madea, B. (2014). *Handbook of Forensic Medicine.* Hoboken, NJ: John Wiley & Sons, p. 49.

4 DiMaio, V.J. & DiMaio, D. (2001). *Forensic Pathology* (second edition). Boca Raton, FL: CRC Press, p. 1.

5 Ibid..

6 Smith, S. (1951). The history and development of forensic medicine. *British Medical Journal* 1: 599–607.

7 Vieira, D.N. (2008). Foreword. In B. Madea & P. Saukko (eds). *Forensic Medicine in Europe.* Lübeck: Schmidt-Römhild, pp. 13–15.

8 Conan Doyle, A. (1981). *The Celebrated Cases of Sherlock Holmes.* London: Octopus Books, p. 623.

9 Wright, R.K. & Tate, L.G. Forensic pathology: Last stronghold of the autopsy. *American Journal of Forensic Medicine and Pathology* 1(1): 57–60.

10 Madea, B. (2000). Estimation of the time since death. In J.A. Siegel & P.J. Saukko (eds). *Encyclopedia of Forensic Sciences.* Volume 3. Amsterdam: Elsevier, pp. 229–237. See also DiMaio, V.J. & DiMaio, D. (2001). *Forensic Pathology* (second edition). Boca Raton, FL: CRC Press, pp. 21–41.

11 The International Coalition against Enforced Disappearances, which gathers family member organisations and human rights organisations from around the world, joins hands for a global event to promote the ratification of the International Convention for the Protection of All Persons from Enforced Disappearance.

12 Capstick, P.H. (1978). *Death in the Long Grass: A Big Game Hunter's Adventures in the African Bush.* New York, NY: St Martin's Press.

13 Pearse, R.O. & Byrom, J. (1990). *Dragon's Wrath: Drakensberg Climbs, Accidents and Rescues.* Midrand: Southern Book Publishers.

14 Silva, L.M.A., Cooper, M.A., Blumenthal, R. & Pliskin, N. (2016). A follow-up study of a large group of children struck by lightning. *South African Medical Journal* 106(9): 929–932.

15 William, M. (2013). Cape buffalo sold for R40m – PIC. IOL, 19 September 2013. Available at https://www.iol.co.za/news/south-africa/limpopo/cape-buffalo-sold-for-r40m-pic-1580001

16 Alexander, M.E., Mutch, R.W., Davis, K.M. & Bucks, C.M. (2017). Wildland fires: Dangers and survival. In P.S. Auerbach (ed.). *Auerbach's Wilderness Medicine*. Volume 1 (seventh edition). Amsterdam: Elsevier, pp. 276–318.

17 Payne-James, J., Jones, R., Karch, S.B. & Manlove, J. (2011). *Simpson's Forensic Medicine* (thirteenth edition). London: Hodder Arnold, p. 216.

18 UNAIDS. (2019). *Global HIV and AIDS statistics: 2019 fact sheet*. Available at https://www.unaids.org/en/resources/fact-sheet

19 Wilkins, D., Woolcock, A.J. & Cossart, Y.E. (1994). Tuberculosis: Medical students at risk. *Medical Journal of Australia* 160(7): 395–397.

20 Templeton, G.L., Illing, L.A., Young, L., Cave, D., Stead, W.W. & Bates, J.H. (1995). The risk for transmission of *Mycobacterium tuberculosis* at the bedside and during autopsy. *Annals of Internal Medicine* 122(12): 922–925.

21 Prusiner, S.B. (1997). Prion diseases and the BSE crisis. *Science* 278(5336): 245–251.

22 Miller, D.C. (1988). Creutzfeldt–Jakob disease in histopathology technicians. *New England Journal of Medicine* 318(13): 853–854.

23 Clayton, S.M. (1993). The high-risk autopsy: Recognition and protection. *American Journal of Forensic Medicine and Pathology* 14(3): 253–256.

24 Al-Wali, A. (2001). Biological safety. In J.L Burton & G.N. Rutty (eds). *The Hospital Autopsy*. London: Arnold, pp. 25–36.

25 Fineschi ,V., Aprile, A., Aquila, I., et al. (2020). Management of the corpse with suspect, probable or confirmed COVID-19 respiratory infection – Italian interim recommendations for personnel potentially exposed to material from corpses, including body fluids, in morgue structures and during autopsy practice. *Pathologica*, 26 March 2020.

26 Montaro, A. (1996). Formaldehyde in the workplace and in the home: Exploring its clinical toxicology. *Laboratory Medicine* 27(11): 752–758.

27 Salkie, M.L. (1991). The prevalence of atopy and hypersensitivity to formaldehyde in pathologists. *Archives of Pathology and Laboratory Medicine* 115(6): 614–616.

28 Sterling, T.D. & Weinkam, J.J. (1988). Reanalysis of lung cancer mortality in a National Cancer Institute study on mortality among industrial workers exposed to formaldehyde. *Journal of Occupational Medicine* 30(11): 895–901.

29 Andrews, J.M., Sweeney, E.S., Grey, T.C. & Wetzel, T. (1989). The bio-
    hazard potential of cyanide poisoning during postmortem examination.
    Journal of Forensic Sciences 34(5): 1280–1284.

30 Copeland, A.R. (1988). Organophosphate related fatalities – a violitional
    biohazard? *Forensic Science International* 39(2): 155–162.

31 Sidell, F.R. (1997). Nerve agents. In F.R. Sidell, E.T. Takafuji & D.R.
    Franz (eds). *Medical Aspects of Chemical and Biological Warfare*. Washing-
    ton, DC: Borden Institute, Walter Reed Army Medical Center, pp. 129–179.

32 St. Germain, J. (1986). The radioactive patient. *Seminars in Nuclear
    Medicine* 16(3): 179–183.

33 Simkins, H., Fink, L.M. & Prasad, K. (1977). Radioisotopes in tissues of
    patients studied at autopsy. *New England Journal of Medicine* 296 (8): 456.

34 Prahlow, J.A., Guileyardo, J.M. & Barnard, J.J. (1997). The implantable
    cardioverter-defibrillator: A potential hazard for pathologists. *Archives
    of Pathology and Laboratory Medicine* 121(10): 1076–1080.

35 Mason, J.K. & Purdue, B.N. (2000). *The Pathology of Trauma* (third edi-
    tion). London: Arnold, pp. 235–236.

36 Schwär, T.G., Loubser, J.D. & Olivier, J.A. (1998). *The Forensic ABC in
    Medical Practice: A practical guide*. Pretoria: Haum Educational Publish-
    ers, pp. 68–71.

37 Simpson C.K. (1965). *Taylor's Principles and Practice of Medical Juris-
    prudence* (12th edition). London: J and A Churchill. See also Mason,
    J.K. and Purdue B.N. (200). *The Pathology of Trauma* (3rd edition).
    Arnold Publishers, p. 235.

38 Kumar P., Rayamane A.P., Subbaramaiah M. Sudden death due to
    Eagle syndrome: A case report. *American Journal of Forensic Medicine
    and Pathology*. 2013; 34(3):231-233. doi:10.1097/PAF.0b013e3182a186e1

39 Mason, J.K. & Purdue, B.N. (2000). *The Pathology of Trauma* (third edi-
    tion). London: Arnold, pp. 235–236.

40 Payne-James, J. & Jones, R. (2020). *Simpson's Forensic Medicine* (four-
    teenth edition). Boca Raton, FL: CRC Press, pp. 261–263.

41 Srisont, S., Chirachariyavej, T. & Peonim, A.V. (2009). A carbon dioxide
    fatality from dry ice. *Journal of Forensic Sciences* 54(4): 961–962.

42 Morris, D. (1999). *Body Guards: Protective Amulets and Charms*. London:
    Element Books.

43 Schwär, T.G., Loubser, J.D. & Olivier, J.A. (1988). *The Forensic ABC in
    Medical Practice: A practical guide*. Pretoria: Haum Educational Pub-
    lishers.

44 Sackner-Bernstein, J. (2017). Design of hack-resistant diabetes devices and
    disclosure of their cyber safety. *Journal of Diabetes Science and Technology*

11(2): 198–202. See also Khera, M. (2017). Think like a hacker: Insights on the latest attack vectors (and security controls) for medical device applications. *Journal of Diabetes Science and Technology* 11(2): 207–212.

45 University of Leicester. (2008). Criminals who eat processed foods more likely to be discovered, through fingerprint sweat corroding metal. *ScienceDaily*, 18 September 2008. See also David T.J., Ajdukiewicz, A.B. & Read, A.E. (1970). Fingerprint changes in coeliac disease. *British Medical Journal* 4(5735): 594–596 and Cherill, F.A. (1950). Fingerprints and disease. *Nature* 166: 581.

46 Macoveciuc, I., Rando, C.J. & Borrion, H. (2019). Forensic gait analysis and recognition: Standards of evidence admissibility. *Journal of Forensic Science* 64(5): 1294–1303.

47 Jones, B.J. & Kenyon, A.J. (2008). Retention of data in heat-damaged SIM cards and potential recovery methods. *Forensic Science International* 177(1): 42–46.

48 Payne-James, J. & Jones, R. (2020). *Simpson's Forensic Medicine* (fourteenth edition). Boca Raton, FL: CRC Press, pp. 86–87.

49 Bright, F.M., Vink, R., Byard, R.W., Duncan, J.R., Krous, H.F. & Paterson, D.S. (2017). Abnormalities in substance P neurokinin-1 receptor binding in key brainstem nuclei in sudden infant death syndrome related to prematurity and sex. *PLoS ONE* 12(9): e0184958. See also Paterson, D.S., Trachtenberg, F.L., Thompson, E.G., et al. (2006). Multiple serotonergic brainstem abnormalities in sudden infant death syndrome. JAMA 296(17): 2124–2132.

50 Garriott, J.C. (2009). *Garriott's Medicolegal Aspects of Alcohol* (fifth edition). Tucson, AZ: Lawyers & Judges Publishing Company, Inc., pp. 434–436.

51 Watch a video on Scarpetta House at https://www.youtube.com/watch?v=gCCzcpaXXbU

52 Taleb, N.N. (2018). *Skin in the Game*. New York, NY: Random House, p. 141.

53 Bokser, B.Z. (2001). *The Wisdom of the Talmud*. New York, NY: Citadel Press, p. 157.

54 Balachandran, A., Krishnan, B. & John, L. (2013). Accidental deaths due to electrocution during amateur electro-fishing. *Journal of Evolution of Medical and Dental Sciences* 2(48): 9376–9379.

55 Chophi, R., Sharma, S., Sharma, S. & Singh, R. (2019). Trends in the forensic analysis of cosmetic evidence. *Forensic Chemistry* 14: 100165

56 Frankl, V.E. (1947). *Man's Search for Meaning* (second edition). Boston, MA: Beacon Press (English).

57 Knight, B. (1996). *Forensic Pathology* (second edition). London: Arnold.

58 Dolinak, D. & Balraj, E.K. (2006). In Memoriam: Lester Adelson, MD
    (1914–2006). *American Journal of Forensic Medicine and Pathology* 27(3):
    283–284.

59 Ibid.

60 Ibid.

61 Levitan, A.A. (1985). Hypnotic death rehearsal. *American Journal of
    Clinical Hypnosis* 27(4): 211–215.

62 The dead open the eyes of the living, or *i morti verze i oci ai vivi*, is a
    Venetian proverb.

63 Dolinak, D. & Balraj, E.K. (2006). In Memoriam: Lester Adelson, MD
    (1914–2006). *American Journal of Forensic Medicine and Pathology* 27(3):
    283–284.

64 Wright, R.K. & Tate, L.G. (1980). Forensic pathology. Last stronghold
    of the autopsy. *American Journal of Forensic Medicine and Pathology* 1(1):
    57–60.

About the author

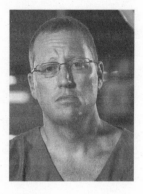 RYAN BLUMENTHAL, MBChB (Pret), MMed (Med Forens) Pret, FC For Path (SA), Dip For Med (SA), PhD (Wits) is a forensic pathologist based in South Africa.

He has published widely in the fields of electrocution, suicide and other areas involving the pathology of trauma. His chief mission in life is to help advance forensic pathology services both nationally and internationally.

Photo: E de Pauw and D Fisher (Walla Films)